Quick & Easy
LOW CHOLESTEROL RECIPES
for Beginners

Quarto.com

© 2024 Quarto Publishing Group USA Inc.
Text © 2009 Dick Logue

First Published in 2024 by New Shoe Press, an imprint of The Quarto Group,
100 Cummings Center, Suite 265-D, Beverly, MA 01915, USA.
T (978) 282-9590 F (978) 283-2742

Essential, In-Demand Topics, Four-Color Design, Affordable Price
New Shoe Press publishes affordable, beautifully designed books covering evergreen, in-demand subjects. With a goal to inform and inspire readers' everyday hobbies, from cooking and gardening to wellness and health to art and crafts, New Shoe titles offer the ultimate library of purposeful, how-to guidance aimed at meeting the unique needs of each reader. Reimagined and redesigned from Quarto's best-selling backlist, New Shoe books provide practical knowledge and opportunities for all DIY enthusiasts to enrich and enjoy their lives.

Visit Quarto.com/New-Shoe-Press for a complete listing of the New Shoe Press books.

New Shoe Press titles are also available at discount for retail, wholesale, promotional, and bulk purchase. For details, contact the Special Sales Manager by email at specialsales@quarto.com or by mail at The Quarto Group, Attn: Special Sales Manager, 100 Cummings Center, Suite 265-D, Beverly, MA 01915, USA.

10 9 8 7 6 5 4 3 2 1

ISBN: 978-0-7603-9056-6
eISBN: 978-0-7603-9057-3

The content in this book was previously published in 500 Low Cholesterol Recipes (Fair Winds Press 2009) by Dick Logue.

Library of Congress Cataloging-in-Publication Data available

Printed in China

The information in this book is for educational purposes only. It is not intended to replace the advice of a physician or medical practitioner. Please see your health-care provider before beginning any new health program.

Quick & Easy
LOW CHOLESTEROL RECIPES
for Beginners

Flavorful Heart-Healthy Dishes Your Whole Family Will Love

DICK LOGUE

NEW SHOE PRESS

Dedication

To my wife, Ginger DeMarco, who has supported
me through the good recipes and the failures.

Contents

What Is This Cholesterol Thing Anyway?

These days it seems like the topic of lowering your cholesterol is on everyone's lips. You see articles about it in your local newspaper and ads for medications on TV, and it's become a common topic of conversation. Perhaps you are looking at this book because your doctor told you your cholesterol was "high" or "borderline." It seems that terms like these are thrown out all the time. Perhaps you already have other heart or vascular problems that can be aggravated by elevated cholesterol. Or perhaps you're just trying to eat a heart-healthy diet.

Whatever the reason, you probably have questions like:

- What is cholesterol, and how high does it have to be to be a problem?
- What's all this talk about good and bad cholesterol?
- What kind of changes do I need to make to my diet and lifestyle to lower my cholesterol?
- Who are you and why are you writing this book?

In this introduction, we're going to try to answer some of those questions. We'll look at lowering your cholesterol primarily from a dietary standpoint because, after all, this is a cookbook. But I'll also mention some of the other things that can also help. What I'm not going to do is give you medical advice. You should always talk to your doctor or other health care provider if you have medical questions.

A Quick Basic Course in Cholesterol

To start, let's see if we can come up with a simple explanation of what cholesterol is and how it affects our health. Cholesterol is a fatty substance that exists in all of our bodies. Some of our organs, like the brain and the heart, actually need cholesterol to perform their functions. It travels through the body in the bloodstream and is processed by the liver. So far, that's not a problem. The problem comes when we have excess cholesterol. It can attach itself to the walls of our blood vessels, forming a substance called plaque, which is really just cholesterol that the body stores in a blood vessel and is covered over with a protective coating. But there are several problems with that. One is that the plaque can build up to the point where it can block a blood vessel. This can cause a restriction of blood flow to important organs like the heart and the brain. The other problem occurs if the coating gets broken and the cholesterol gets released back into the bloodstream. This causes the body to send chemicals that help the blood to clot to try and get the cholesterol back under cover and can cause a blood clot. If that clot blocks an artery in the heart, that's what we call a heart attack. If it happens in the brain, that's a stroke.

The next question is what causes us to have high cholesterol. As you've probably heard in the advertisements on television, cholesterol is caused both by genetic factors and your diet. If your parents or grandparents had high cholesterol, the chances increase that you will too. The one thing doctors don't know at this point is whether that elevated risk is caused entirely by genetics or whether people whose parents had bad eating habits tend to eat the same way, meaning that even the hereditary risk may still be caused partly by diet. What we do know is that diet plays a major part in determining cholesterol levels. And the biggest culprit in our diets is saturated fats. Unfortunately, a lot of the things that we like to eat are high in saturated fats, such as fatty meats; fried foods; high-fat dairy products like whole milk, cream, and cheese made from whole milk; and commercial baked products. As we get into the recipes in this book, we'll look at some alternatives that are lower in saturated fats, but still taste good.

What about This Good and Bad Cholesterol?

When your doctor does a blood test to check your cholesterol levels, he's looking for a couple of different things. These are subcomponents of cholesterol, and they are not at all the same in terms of your health. The three primary ones most often tested for are low-density lipo-proteins (LDL), high-density lipoproteins (HDL), and triglycerides. The levels of these cholesterol components are measured in mg/dl, the number of milligrams of the substance in a deciliter of blood. Let take a quick look at each of them.

LDL is commonly referred to as bad cholesterol. It is the part of your total cholesterol that plays the biggest role in blocking your arteries. When LDL attaches to an artery wall, it causes an inflammation that encourages more cholesterol to be deposited there, increasing the risk of a blockage or blood clot. Eating foods high in saturated fats is a major cause of an increase in LDL. The level of LDL that poses a risk is still a subject of discussion, but everyone agrees that anything over 200 mg/dl is dangerous. Some doctors believe that, depending on the source and on what other risk factors (like smoking and being overweight) you may have, even levels over 100 mg/dl may increase your risk of heart attack and stroke.

HDL is usually called the good cholesterol. HDL helps the body rid itself of the cholesterol deposits in the arteries. A high HDL level indicates that you probably have a low risk of heart attack. It has been recommended that men have an HDL of at least 40 mg/dl and women at least 50 mg/dl. The good news is that doing the things that lower your LDL tend to raise your HDL levels. And adding good fat to your diet helps to raise HDL. Some sources are fatty fish like tuna and salmon, olive and canola oil, and the oils found in nuts and soybeans. Some studies even suggest that a moderate amount of alcohol will raise your HDL.

The third major component of a typical cholesterol screening is triglycerides. Like LDL, triglycerides can contribute to a buildup of deposits in the arteries. And like LDL, they are raised by a diet high in saturated fats. It's recommended that triglyceride levels be less than 150 mg/dl.

It should probably be noted that a number of doctors believe that the ratio between HDL and LDL is even more important than the individual numbers. So anything we do to lower our LDL or raise our HDL has a positive effect on that ratio.

How Do I Lower My Cholesterol?

As we've seen, there are a number of factors that contribute to your cholesterol and overall heart health. Some of them, like genetics and age, we have no control over. But others we do. When it comes down to it, there are three main things we can do to lower cholesterol. One is medication, and that is something to take up with your doctor. Another is exercise. Studies have shown that regular exercise can lower cholesterol and reduce the risk of heart disease and stroke. My cardiologist recommends 30 minutes of walking a day as a minimum. It isn't all that difficult, but it does take a commitment.

The final factor is diet. And that is the reason for this book. There are a couple of things we can do from a dietary standpoint that will help. The first thing, which goes hand in hand with exercise, is to maintain your proper body weight. Being overweight is a known risk factor for heart disease.

The second, as mentioned earlier, is to limit the amount of saturated fat in your diet. The good news is that nutrition labels are now required to list the amount of saturated fat, so it's fairly easy to keep track of. But saturated fat isn't the only bad fat. There are also trans fatty acids, or trans fats, which are produced by hydrogenating liquid fat to make it solid at room temperature, like in making margarine. Trans fats are now also listed on the nutrition labels of packaged foods, making them easier to track. If trans fats are not given in the nutritional information, such as in a recipe, you can easily calculate them by taking the total fat and subtracting the saturated fat, monounsaturated fat, and polyunsaturated fat that are listed. That is also true of the nutrition information in this book. In general, any solid fat is bad fat. Also bad are tropical oils like coconut and palm oil. One rule of thumb is that that you should consume no more than 10 percent of your calories per day from saturated fats and trans fats. Since each gram of fat contains about 100 calories, that makes the calculation fairly easy. If you are eating 2,000 calories a day (the number used as a reference on nutrition labels), then 200 of those calories, at the most, should come from saturated fats and trans fat. That would be 20 grams of bad fats per day maximum.

There are also positive diet changes that you can make. Let's take a quick look at some of them here. We'll go into a more detail in Chapter 1 about how to get them into your diet.

Olive and Canola Oils

While we want to limit the amount of fats in our diet to help us maintain our ideal weight, oils like olive and canola can actually help lower cholesterol. They contain polyunsaturated fat, which is the most healthful kind. All of the recipes in this book that contain oil specify either olive or canola.

Fish

The oils in fish contain a compound called omega-3 fatty acids that help reduce blood vessel blockages and clots. Medical experts often recommend that you eat fish at least twice a week.

Soy

Soy protein, such as that found in tofu, soybeans, and soy-based dairy substitutes, contains compounds that encourage blood vessels to dilate effectively so they can supply the blood needed by the body. It also contains antioxidants, which have been shown to help lower the incidence of cancer and heart disease.

Nuts

Like fish, nuts contain omega-3 fatty acids. They are high in calories, though, so you should eat them in moderation.

Oats and Other Whole Grains

Oats and whole grains contain a number of nutrients that are removed from refined grain products like white flour. Oats also contains water-soluble fiber, which has been proven in a number of studies to reduce LDL cholesterol levels without also lowering the HDL levels. Other foods containing significant soluble fiber include beans, barley, and wheat bran.

How This Book Came About

Perhaps the best way to start in telling you who I am is by telling you who I'm not. I'm not a doctor. I'm not a dietician. I'm not a professional chef. What I *am* is an ordinary person just like you who has some special dietary needs. What I am going to do is give you 500 recipes that I have made for myself and my family that I think will put you on the right track to beating high cholesterol through diet. Many of them are the kind of things people cook in their own kitchens all the time, but modified to make them healthier without losing the flavor.

I've enjoyed cooking most of my life. I guess I started seriously about the time my mother went back to work when I was 12 or so. In those days, it was simple stuff like burgers and hot dogs and spaghetti. But the interest stayed. After I married my wife, we got pretty involved in some food-related stuff like growing vegetables in our garden, making bread and other baked goods, canning and jelly making, that kind of thing. She always said that my "mad chemist" cooking was an outgrowth of the time I spent in college as a chemistry major, and she might be right.

Some of you may already know me from my Low Sodium Cooking website and newsletter, or from my *500 Low Sodium Recipes* book. I started thinking about low sodium cooking after being diagnosed with congestive heart failure in 1999. One of the first, and biggest, things I had to deal with was the doctor's insistence that I follow a low sodium diet: 1,200 mg a day or less. At first, I found it easiest just to avoid the things that had a lot of sodium in them. But I was bored. I was convinced that there had to be a way to create low sodium versions of the foods I missed. I researched where to get low sodium substitutes for the things that I couldn't have any more, bought cookbooks, and basically re-did my whole diet.

Along the way, I learned some things. So I decided to try to share this information with others who may in the same position I had been in. I started a website, www.lowsodiumcooking.com, to share recipes and information. I sent out an email newsletter with recipes that now has over 17,000 subscribers. And I wrote my first book.

Everything was going along well. Then the doctor mentioned that my cholesterol had been creeping up and was now at a level where I should start to make some dietary modifications. All of a sudden, the recipes I had weren't what I needed anymore. I'd been using unsalted butter because it was easy to find and tasty. No more, too much saturated fat. The same with eggs and all the fried food and red meat we'd come to love. So it was back to the kitchen to create more recipes, ones that would be low cholesterol as well as low sodium. This book is the result.

How Is the Nutritional Information Calculated?

The nutritional information included with these recipes was calculated using the AccuChef program. It calculates the values using the latest U.S. Department of Agriculture Standard reference nutritional database. I've been using this program since I first started trying to figure out how much sodium was in the recipes I've created. It's inexpensive, easy to use, and has a number of really handy features. AccuChef is available online from www.accuchef.com. They offer a free trial version if you want to try it out, and the full version costs less than $20 USD.

Of course, that implies that these figures are estimates. Every brand of canned tomatoes, or any other product, is a little different in nutritional content. These figures were calculated using products that I buy where I live in southern Maryland. If you use a different brand, your nutrition figures may be different. Use the nutritional analysis as a guideline in determining whether a recipe is right for your diet.

Saturated Fats

Saturated fats are a primary culprit in raising your cholesterol level. In general, saturated fats are fats that are solid at room temperature. There are several categories of saturated fats, and the amount of saturated fat is listed on the U.S. nutrition facts label on packaged foods. This means that *you* are in control of how much saturated fat you eat. A general recommendation from the American Heart Association and others is to limit yourself to no more than 20 grams of saturated fat a day. The recipes in this book will point the way to the cuts of meat and the cooking techniques that will let you meet that goal.

Red Meats

Beef, pork, and lamb are often considered the worst in terms of saturated fat. It's true that they tend to have more than fish or poultry. But how much they have is very dependent on which cut you choose. Some high-fat cuts of beef may contain five times the amount of saturated fat as a lean cut.

Poultry Skin

While not containing as much saturated fat as red meat, poultry skin does have a significant amount. A chicken thigh with the skin has more than 2 grams additional saturated fat compared to the meat only. And this is a case where eliminating that fat is really easy—just don't eat the skin.

Whole-Milk Dairy

Dairy products are another area where making smart choices can significantly reduce the amount of saturated fat. Avoid using products made from whole milk or cream. Choose skim milk, reduced-fat cheeses, and fat-free versions of sour cream and cream cheese. Use fat-free evaporated milk in place of cream.

Tropical Oils

Some plant oils in this category also contain saturated fats. These include palm, palm kernel, and coconut oils, and cocoa butter. They are generally easy to avoid, but be aware that some commercial baked goods and processed foods may contain them.

Trans Fats

Trans fats are also called trans-fatty acids. They are produced by adding hydrogen to vegetable oil through a process called hydrogenation. This makes the fat more solid and less likely to spoil. Although increased awareness of their health risks have started to reduce their use, trans fats are still a common ingredient in commercial baked goods and fried foods. Food manufacturers are required to list trans fat content on nutrition labels. Amounts less than 0.5 grams per serving can be listed as 0 grams trans fat on the food label.

Margarine and Other Hydrogenated Oils

Avoid margarine and solid shortening containing hydrogenated or partially hydrogenated oils. You will see a few recipes in this book that call for margarine where the texture of the food requires solid fat, but in general use liquid or soft margarines whenever possible. We have come to use butter spray bottles, such as I Can't Believe It's Not Butter! Original Buttery Spray, almost exclusively for "buttering" bread and vegetables.

Commercial Baked Goods and Fried Foods

Read ingredient labels and be aware that hydrogenated oils are a common ingredient in commercial baked goods. Even though awareness has increased and many restaurants now fry in oils without trans fats, make sure that you know what you are eating.

Foods Containing Cholesterol

Your body makes all of the cholesterol it needs, but you also get cholesterol from animal products, such as meat, seafood, eggs, and dairy products. While some experts now believe that the amount of cholesterol you eat is less a factor in raised cholesterol levels than was once thought, they still recommend that adults limit their cholesterol intake to 300 mg per day.

Egg Yolks

An egg yolk contains 214 mg of cholesterol, more than two-thirds of the daily maximum recommendation. The good news is that, other than deviled eggs and eggs fried over-easy, I've not found anywhere that you can't use the egg substitute made primarily from egg whites instead of whole eggs. I've even made egg salad by microwaving some, chopping it up, and adding mayonnaise and mustard.

Organ Meats

Beef liver contains over 300 mg of cholesterol per serving; other kinds of liver and organ meats contain similar amounts. I admit I was one of those people who liked liver, but I don't eat it any more.

Shellfish

Shrimp contains over 130 mg of cholesterol per 3-ounce serving. Other shellfish also tends to be higher than meats and fish. I love shellfish, but we now only have it about once a month.

Healthy Oils

When choosing fats, the best choices are monounsaturated and polyunsaturated fats. These fats have been shown to lower your risk of heart disease by reducing the total and LDL (bad) cholesterol levels in your blood.

Monounsaturated Oils

Monounsaturated fats are the healthiest kind. Replace other fats in your diet with them as often as possible. They are usually liquid at room temperature and begin to solidify when refrigerated. Examples are olive, canola, and peanut oils, and the fat found in avocados. The recipes in this book generally use olive oil for cooking and canola oil for baking.

Polyunsaturated Oils

While not having quite the benefits of monounsaturated oils, polyunsaturated oils are still a much better choice than saturated fats and trans fats. They are usually liquid at both room temperature and in the refrigerator and tend to become rancid if stored too long unrefrigerated. Examples are safflower, sesame, soy, corn, and sunflower-seed oils, and the oils in nuts and seeds.

Foods Containing Omega-3 Fatty Acids

One particular kind of polyunsaturated fat, omega-3 fatty acids, may be especially good for your heart. Omega-3 fatty acids appear to decrease the risk of coronary artery disease.

Fish

Recent dietary recommendations usually call for one or two servings of fish a week. Fortunately, fish lends itself to many kinds of recipes. You'll find a number of fish recipes in this book to get you started. Some are specific to one kind of fish, like tuna steaks, but many can be adapted to use whatever you have on hand or find at a good price.

Nuts

Nuts can be added to many foods to give a little extra boost of omega-3s. While they don't contain as much as fish, they are still a healthy addition. Consider using them as salad toppings rather than bacon bits, stir them into baked goods, or add them to your breakfast cereal.

Flaxseed and Soybeans

I have to admit that I've not tried adding flaxseed to recipes. It does contain omega-3 fatty acids, but not the same levels as fish and nuts. We *have* added more soy to our diet, though, finding not only that tofu is good stir-fried, but also that it works great as a substitute for cheese in things like lasagna and enchiladas. You'll find some good tofu recipes scattered throughout this book.

Foods Containing Whole Grains and Soluble Fiber

Soluble fiber has been shown to lower total cholesterol and LDL without affecting the good cholesterol (HDL).

Oats

Oats have certainly gotten the most notice for their cholesterol-fighting abilities. The U.S. Food and Drug Administration was convinced enough to allow medical claims of cholesterol reduction on packages of oatmeal and oat bran. You can easily add oat bran to many foods, such as breading mixes for meat, as well as the more common baked goods. I've included a number of recipes here that include oat bran. The manufacturers of oatmeal and oat bran also provide lots of information on how to include more of their products in your diet.

Beans and Barley

Dried beans and peas contain a significant amount of soluble fiber. So do grains like barley. These products can also help you cut back on saturated fats by being the basis of meals containing little or no meat. Often they are used in soups and stews, and you'll find a variety of recipes here that include them.

Whole Grains

Experts knew that whole grains are healthier than refined grains long before the benefits of soluble fiber were understood. In many cases, it's an easy switch to choose whole-grain products like bread, rice, and pasta rather than their refined counterparts. The great news is that some people find they also taste better.

Fruits and Vegetables

Some fruits and vegetables contain enough soluble fiber to provide benefits. The most common are apples, strawberries, oranges, bananas, carrots, corn, cauliflower, and sweet potatoes.

How Can We Make Our Diets Healthier?

So what did I really do to make my diet healthier than the way I used to eat? In general, here are the guidelines I followed:

- Reduce saturated fats as much as possible by making healthy ingredient choices. Limit the number of servings of red meat each week, and choose lean cuts when it is on the menu. Choose fat-free or reduced-fat dairy products whenever available. Avoiding using tropical oils that contain saturated fat.

- Avoid using trans fats as much as possible. Use olive oil for cooking and canola oil for baking in place of other fats.

- Reduce your total fat intake. While some fats are healthier than others and do provide benefits, it is still recommended that less than 10 percent of your total calories come from fat. Reduce consumption of fried foods and high-fat baked goods. Replace some or all of the fat in baked goods with fruit.

- Avoid whole eggs. Use egg substitute in place of whole eggs wherever possible.

- Reduce consumption of other foods with high cholesterol levels, particularly organ meats and shellfish.

- Increase consumption of omega-3 fatty acids. Eat more fish. Adds nuts to baked goods and salads for an extra omega-3 boost.

- Add more whole grains to your diet. Eat whole-grain breads and other baked goods. Replace white rice with brown. Choose whole-grain pastas over regular.

- Increase the amount of other soluble fiber in your diet. Eat more oat bran, beans, and barley.

Where's the Salt?

One question that may occur to some people looking over the recipes in this book is, "Why is there no salt in any of the ingredient lists?" That's a fair question and deserves an answer. As I said in the Introduction, I first got involved with heart-healthy cooking because my doctor put me on a low sodium diet. It took some time and lots of experimentation, but I learned how to cook things that taste good, are easy to prepare, and are still low in sodium. Along the way, we literally threw away our saltshaker. There's one shaker full of light salt (half salt and half salt substitute) on the table. My wife uses that occasionally. Two of my children have given up salt completely, not because they need to for medical reasons, but because they are convinced like I am that it's the healthy thing to do. When I started looking at creating low cholesterol recipes, going back to using salt wasn't even something I considered.

Most Americans get far more than the 2,400 mg of sodium a day recommended for a healthy adult. This happens without our even thinking about it. In creating these recipes, I was not as strict about the amount of sodium as I usually am. I didn't plan on people buying special sodium-free baking powder that is difficult to find except online. I didn't eliminate most cheeses except Swiss. But I also didn't add any salt. I think if you try the recipes, you'll find that they taste good without it. If you are tempted to add some salt because you think it's needed, I'd suggest you check with your cardiologist or other doctor first. I believe that most of them will agree that in the interest of total heart healthiness, you are better off without the salt.

1

Sauces, Condiments, Mixes, and Spice Blends

When you are trying to reduce the amount of fat in your diet, particularly saturated fat, sauces and condiments can be a problem. White sauce? Let's see, that contains 2 tablespoons (28 g) of butter per cup (235 ml) of sauce, right? Not anymore. This chapter contains some tasty, low fat sauces that you can use in your everyday dishes. It also includes a smattering of other things. There are a couple of low fat baking mixes to use in place of commercial mixes and some condiments that are heart-healthier than anything you can find in the store. And, finally, there are a few spice blends for grilling. While these aren't exactly cholesterol-reducing themselves, perhaps they'll encourage you to try some of the grilling and smoking recipes. These methods of cooking are good for reducing the amount of fat in your final dish, since it's allowed to drip away during the cooking process.

Tomato and Avocado Salsa

Can't make up your mind if you want salsa or guacamole? Then have both together!

5 plum tomatoes

¼ cup (40 g) red onion, diced

1 jalapeño, seeded and chopped

1 avocado, diced

2 tablespoons (30 ml) lime juice

1 tablespoon (4 g) cilantro

Halve the tomatoes and remove the seeds, then chop fi nely. Put into a bowl with other ingredients. Stir to mix.

—
Yield: 8 servings

PER SERVING: 34 calories (65% from fat, 6% from protein, 30% from carbohydrate); 1 g protein; 3 g total fat; 0 g saturated fat; 2 g monounsaturated fat; 0 g polyunsaturated fat; 3 g carbohydrate; 1 g fiber; 1 g sugar; 14 mg phosphorus; 5 mg calcium; 0 mg iron; 2 mg sodium; 125 mg potassium; 140 IU vitamin A; 0 mg ATE vitamin E; 5 mg vitamin C; 0 mg cholesterol; 31 g water

Reduced-Sodium Soy Sauce

Even though sodium is not directly tied to cholesterol, it is definitely connected to heart health. Soy sauce, even the reduced-sodium kinds, contains more sodium than many people's diets can stand. A teaspoonful often contains at least a quarter of the daily amount of sodium that is recommended for a healthy adult. If you have heart disease or are African American, the recommendation is even less. This sauce gives you real soy sauce flavor while holding the sodium to a level that should fit in most people's diets.

4 tablespoons (24 g) sodium-free beef bouillon

¼ cup (60 ml) cider vinegar

2 tablespoons (30 ml) molasses

1½ cups (355 ml) boiling water

⅛ teaspoon (0.3 g) black pepper

⅛ teaspoon (0.2 g) ground ginger

¼ teaspoon (0.8 g) garlic powder

¼ cup (60 ml) reduced-sodium soy sauce

Combine ingredients, stirring to blend thoroughly. Pour into jars. Cover and seal tightly. Keeps indefinitely if refrigerated.

—
Yield: 48 servings

PER SERVING: 6 calories (13% from fat, 11% from protein, 76% from carbohydrate); 0 g protein; 0 g total fat; 0 g saturated fat; 0 g monounsaturated fat; 0 g polyunsaturated fat; 1 g carbohydrate; 0 g fiber; 1 g sugar; 3 mg phosphorus; 4 mg calcium; 0 mg iron; 52 mg sodium; 19 mg potassium; 3 IU vitamin A; 0 mg ATE vitamin E; 0 mg vitamin C; 0 mg cholesterol; 10 g water

Reduced-Sodium Teriyaki Sauce

The story on this recipe is the same as the soy sauce. In this case, you can sometimes find commercial teriyaki sauces that aren't too high in sodium, but this one is much lower and, to my mind, tastes just as good, if not better.

1 cup (235 ml) Reduced-Sodium Soy Sauce (see recipe page 15)

1 tablespoon (15 ml) sesame oil

2 tablespoons (30 ml) mirin wine

½ cup (100 g) sugar

2 cloves garlic, crushed

Two ⅛-inch (31-mm) slices ginger root

Dash black pepper

Combine all ingredients in a saucepan and heat until the sugar is dissolved. Store in the refrigerator.

—
Yield: 20 servings

PER SERVING: 37 calories (2% from fat, 0% from protein, 98% from carbohydrate); 0 g protein; 1 g total fat; 0 g saturated fat; 0 g monounsaturated fat; 2 g polyunsaturated fat; 84 g carbohydrate; 0 g fiber; 7 g sugar; 10 mg phosphorus; 7 mg calcium; 0 mg iron; 83 mg sodium; 32 mg potassium; 5 IU vitamin A; 0 mg ATE vitamin E; 0 mg vitamin C; 0 mg cholesterol; 17 g water

TIP

Mirin is a sweet Japanese rice wine; you can substitute sherry or sake.

Chipotle Marinade

Depending on the peppers you use, this can be hot or not. The ancho chilis are less hot than some. A serving is one tablespoon.

2 ounces (55 g) dried ancho chilis

1 teaspoon (2 g) black pepper

2 teaspoons (4.7 g) cumin

2 tablespoons (8 g) fresh oregano, chopped

1 small red onion, quartered

½ cup (120 ml) lime juice

½ cup (120 ml) cider vinegar

3 cloves garlic, peeled

1 cup (60 g) fresh cilantro

½ cup (120 ml) olive oil

Soak dry chilis in water overnight, or until soft. Remove seeds. Place chilis and remaining ingredients in a food processor or blender and process until smooth.

—
Yield: 32 servings

PER SERVING: 39 calories (79% from fat, 3% from protein, 18% from carbohydrate); 0 g protein; 4 g total fat; 0 g saturated fat; 2 g monounsaturated fat; 0 g polyunsaturated fat; 2 g carbohydrate; 1 g fiber; 0 g sugar; 7 mg phosphorus; 8 mg calcium; 0 mg iron; 2 mg sodium; 67 mg potassium; 467 IU vitamin A; 0 mg ATE vitamin E; 2 mg vitamin C; 0 mg cholesterol; 11 g water

Chipotle Sauce

This creamy sauce can be used in a number of dishes and is traditional for fish tacos.

½ cup (115 g) low fat mayonnaise

½ cup (115 g) fat-free sour cream

¼ cup (60 ml) Chipotle Marinade (see recipe page 32)

Mix ingredients and chill.

—
Yield: 10 servings

PER SERVING: 56 calories (82% from fat, 4% from protein, 14% from carbohydrate); 0 g protein; 4 g total fat; 1 g saturated fat; 0 g monounsaturated fat; 0 g polyunsaturated fat; 2 g carbohydrate; 0 g fiber; 1 g sugar; 18 mg phosphorus; 13 mg calcium; 0 mg iron; 101 mg sodium; 22 mg potassium; 67 IU vitamin A; 12 mg ATE vitamin E; 0 mg vitamin C; 9 mg cholesterol; 16 g water

Bread and Butter Onions

Okay, I admit there isn't really anything about this recipe that is, by itself, good for your cholesterol. But I made a batch of these this summer after seeing them at an Amish stand at the local farmer's market, and I've become fond of them as a condiment with a number of things. They just add a nice little extra bit of flavor.

4 onions

1¼ cups (300 ml) cider vinegar

1¼ cups (250 g) sugar

½ teaspoon (1.1 g) turmeric

½ teaspoon (1.8 g) mustard seed

¼ teaspoon (0.5 g) celery seed

Thinly slice onions and separate into rings. In a saucepan, combine vinegar, sugar, turmeric, mustard seed, and celery seed. Heat to boiling. Add onions. Heat 2 to 3 minutes. Chill and serve. May be stored in the refrigerator for one month. For longer storage, sterilize two pint (475 ml) jars. Pack hot pickles to within ½ inch (1.3 cm) of the top. Wipe off the rim, screw on the lid, and place in a Dutch oven or other deep pan. Cover with hot water, bring to a boil, and cook 5 minutes.

—

Yield: 32 servings

PER SERVING: 41 calories (1% from fat, 2% from protein, 97% from carbohydrate); 0 g protein; 0 g total fat; 0 g saturated fat; 0 g monounsaturated fat; 0 g polyunsaturated fat; 10 g carbohydrate; 0 g fiber; 9 g sugar; 7 mg phosphorus; 6 mg calcium; 0 mg iron; 1 mg sodium; 38 mg potassium; 0 IU vitamin A; 0 mg ATE vitamin E; 1 mg vitamin C; 0 mg cholesterol; 27 g water

Reduced-Fat Biscuit Mix

This makes a mix similar to Reduced Fat Bisquick, but mine is even lower in fat. Use it in any recipes that call for baking mix.

6 cups (750 g) flour

3 tablespoons (41.5 g) baking powder

⅓ cup (75 g) unsalted margarine

Stir flour and baking powder together. Cut in margarine with pastry blender or two knives until mixture resembles coarse crumbs. Store in a container with a tight-fitting lid.

—
Yield: 12 servings

PER SERVING: 274 calories (19% from fat, 10% from protein, 72% from carbohydrate); 7 g protein; 6 g total fat; 1 g saturated fat; 3 g monounsaturated fat; 1 g polyunsaturated fat; 49 g carbohydrate; 2 g fiber; 0 g sugar; 146 mg phosphorus; 216 mg calcium; 3 mg iron; 422 mg sodium; 73 mg potassium; 267 IU vitamin A; 61 mg ATE vitamin E; 0 mg vitamin C; 0 mg cholesterol; 9 g water

Reduced-Fat Whole Wheat Biscuit Mix

I use this mix almost all the time in place of the white flour one.

4 cups (500 g) flour

2 cups (250 g) whole wheat flour

3 tablespoons (41.5 g) baking powder

⅓ cup (75 g) unsalted margarine

Stir flours and baking powder together. Cut in margarine with pastry blender or two knives until mixture resembles coarse crumbs. Store in a container with a tight-fitting lid.

—
Yield: 12 servings

PER SERVING: 266 calories (19% from fat, 11% from protein, 70% from carbohydrate); 7 g protein; 6 g total fat; 1 g saturated fat; 3 g monounsaturated fat; 1 g polyunsaturated fat; 47 g carbohydrate; 4 g fiber; 0 g sugar; 193 mg phosphorus; 220 mg calcium; 3 mg iron; 422 mg sodium; 132 mg potassium; 268 IU vitamin A; 61 mg ATE vitamin E; 0 mg vitamin C; 0 mg cholesterol; 8 g water

The Wild Rub

A traditional southern dry rub for barbecue, typically rubbed into the meat and allowed to flavor it overnight in the refrigerator before long, low heat cooking. The main ingredient is paprika, so if you plan to do a lot of grilling or smoking, you may want to get a big bottle at one of the warehouse clubs like Sam's or BJ's. The rub tends to be a bit on the spicy side, so if you don't like your food hot, you may want to try The Mild Rub (see opposite).

½ cup (56 g) paprika

3 tablespoons (19 g) freshly ground black pepper

¼ cup (60 g) brown sugar

2 tablespoons (15 g) chili powder

2 tablespoons (18 g) onion powder

2 tablespoons (18 g) garlic powder

2 teaspoons (3.6 g) cayenne pepper

Mix well, and store in a cool, dark place.

—
Yield: 22 servings

PER SERVING: 26 calories (15% from fat, 10% from protein, 76% from carbohydrate); 1 g protein; 1 g total fat; 0 g saturated fat; 0 g monounsaturated fat; 0 g polyunsaturated fat; 6 g carbohydrate; 2 g fiber; 3 g sugar; 15 mg calcium; 1 mg iron; 10 mg sodium; 109 mg potassium; 1595 IU vitamin A; 0 mg ATE vitamin E; 3 mg vitamin C; 0 mg cholesterol; 1 g water

The Mild Rub

A sweeter, less spicy rub for grilling and smoking.

½ cup (56 g) paprika

2 tablespoons (13 g) freshly ground black pepper

⅓ cup (75 g) brown sugar

2 tablespoons (15 g) chili powder

2 tablespoons (18 g) onion powder

2 tablespoons (18 g) garlic powder

Mix well, and store in a cool, dark place.

—
Yield: 22 servings

PER SERVING: 28 calories (13% from fat, 9% from protein, 78% from carbohydrate); 1 g protein; 0 g total fat; 0 g saturated fat; 0 g monounsaturated fat; 0 g polyunsaturated fat; 6 g carbohydrate; 1 g fiber; 4 g sugar; 15 mg calcium; 1 mg iron; 10 mg sodium; 105 mg potassium; 1527 IU vitamin A; 0 mg ATE vitamin E; 3 mg vitamin C; 0 mg cholesterol

2

Breakfasts

Breakfast can be another problem time for those of us trying to eat in a cholesterol-friendly way. First, there's the saturated fat in traditional breakfast meats. Then there's the amount of cholesterol in eggs. For those who don't really fancy the idea of granola every day, we have some options. You can easily make sausage that is lower in fat than any you can buy at the store. And egg substitutes, made from egg whites, work fine for omelets, scrambled eggs, and other dishes. As an alternative, there are smoothies, packed with things that are good for you.

Turkey Breakfast Sausage

I've been back at the chemistry table—I mean, kitchen counter—trying various recipes for sausage again. This is my favorite so far. It contains about one twentieth of the sodium, one tenth of the fat, and one third of the calories of the average store-bought sausage.

1 pound (455 g) ground turkey

¼ teaspoon (0.5 g) black pepper

¼ teaspoon (0.5 g) white pepper

¾ teaspoon (0.6 g) dried sage

¼ teaspoon (0.4 g) ground mace

½ teaspoon (1.5 g) garlic powder

¼ teaspoon (0.8 g) onion powder

¼ teaspoon (0.5 g) ground allspice

1 teaspoon (5 ml) olive oil

Combine all ingredients, mixing well. Fry, grill, or preheat oven to 325°F (170°C, or gas mark 3) and cook on a greased baking sheet to desired doneness.

—

Yield: 8 servings

PER SERVING: 69 calories (20% from fat, 77% from protein, 2% from carbohydrate); 13 g protein; 1 g total fat; 0 g saturated fat; 1 g monounsaturated fat; 0 g polyunsaturated fat; 0 g carbohydrate; 0 g fiber; 0 g sugar; 106 mg phosphorus; 9 mg calcium; 1 mg iron; 35 mg sodium; 153 mg potassium; 5 IU vitamin A; 0 mg ATE vitamin E; 0 mg vitamin C; 41 mg cholesterol; 43 g water

Snowy Day Breakfast Casserole

My wife came up with this one winter when we were snowed in. It has since become a standard in our house, just the sort of thing you need when sitting in front of the fire.

2 slices low sodium bacon

3 potatoes, shredded

½ cup (80 g) onion, chopped

¼ cup (37 g) green bell pepper, chopped

1 cup (235 ml) egg substitute

¼ cup (30 g) low fat cheddar cheese, shredded

Preheat oven to 350°F (180°C, or gas mark 4). Fry bacon in a large skillet. Remove bacon to a paper towel–covered plate to drain. Add potatoes, onion, and green pepper to skillet and sauté until potatoes are crispy and onion soft. Stir in crumbled bacon. Transfer to greased 8-inch (20-cm) square baking dish. Pour egg substitute over. Sprinkle with cheese. Bake until eggs are set, about 20 minutes.

—

Yield: 4 servings

PER SERVING: 292 calories (14% from fat, 22% from protein, 63% from carbohydrate); 17 g protein; 5 g total fat; 1 g saturated fat; 1 g monounsaturated fat; 1 g polyunsaturated fat; 47 g carbohydrate; 5 g fiber; 4 g sugar; 314 mg phosphorus; 101 mg calcium; 4 mg iron; 221 mg sodium; 1540 mg potassium; 299 IU vitamin A; 5 mg ATE vitamin E; 33 mg vitamin C; 7 mg cholesterol; 308 g water

Vegetable Omelet

This can be either a breakfast or the main part of an evening meal.

1 tablespoon (15 ml) olive oil

2 ounces (55 g) mushrooms, sliced

¼ cup (40 g) onion, diced

¼ cup (37 g) green bell peppers, diced

¼ cup (28 g) zucchini, sliced

½ cup (90 g) tomato, diced

1 cup (240 ml) egg substitute

2 tablespoons (30 g) fat-free sour cream

2 tablespoons (30 ml) water

2 ounces (55 g) Swiss cheese, shredded

Add olive oil to a large skillet and sauté mushrooms, onion, green bell pepper, zucchini, and tomato until soft, adding tomato last. Whisk together egg substitute, sour cream, and water until fluffy. Coat an omelet pan or skillet with nonstick vegetable spray and place over medium-high heat. Pour egg mixture into pan. Lift the edges as it cooks to allow uncooked egg to run underneath. When eggs are nearly set, cover half the eggs with the cheese and sautéed vegetables and fold the other half over. Continue cooking until eggs are completely set.

—
Yield: 2 servings

PER SERVING: 263 calories (46% from fat, 41% from protein, 13% from carbohydrate); 25 g protein; 13 g total fat; 3 g saturated fat; 6 g monounsaturated fat; 3 g polyunsaturated fat; 8 g carbohydrate; 2 g fiber; 4 g sugar; 386 mg phosphorus; 369 mg calcium; 3 mg iron; 309 mg sodium; 746 mg potassium; 962 IU vitamin A; 26 mg ATE vitamin E; 25 mg vitamin C; 17 mg cholesterol; 259 g water

Sausage Frittata

We like this for breakfast on those rare occasions when the entire family is around, but it also makes a good dinner with a salad and a slice of freshly baked bread.

1 cup (240 ml) egg substitute

¼ cup (60 ml) skim milk

8 ounces (225 g) Turkey Breakfast Sausage (see recipe page 23)

½ cup (75 g) green bell pepper, chopped

4 ounces (115 g) low fat cheddar cheese, shredded

Preheat broiler. Combine egg substitute and milk in medium bowl; whisk until well blended. Set aside. Place a 12-inch (30-cm) broiler-proof nonstick skillet over medium-high heat until hot. Add sausage; cook and stir for 4 minutes or until no longer pink, breaking up sausage with spoon. Drain sausage on paper towels; set aside. Add pepper to same skillet; cook and stir for 2 minutes, or until crisp-tender. Return sausage to skillet. Add egg mixture; stir until blended. Cover; cook over medium-low heat for 10 minutes, or until eggs are almost set. Sprinkle cheese over frittata. Broil for 2 minutes, or until cheese is melted and eggs are set. Cut into wedges.

—
Yield: 4 servings

PER SERVING: 245 calories (54% from fat, 40% from protein, 6% from carbohydrate); 24 g protein; 14 g total fat; 6 g saturated fat; 4 g monounsaturated fat; 3 g polyunsaturated fat; 4 g carbohydrate; 0 g fiber; 1 g sugar; 339 mg phosphorus; 193 mg calcium; 2 mg iron; 626 mg sodium; 398 mg potassium; 385 IU vitamin A; 26 mg ATE vitamin E; 32 mg vitamin C; 41 mg cholesterol; 137 g water

Vegetable Frittata

A frittata is an Italian-style omelet, with the filling mixed in with the eggs. It's cooked without turning and then the top set under the broiler. This version does not have any of the meat and potatoes that they often have, providing you with a filling weekend breakfast low in sodium, fat, and carbohydrates.

½ cup (75 g) red bell pepper, diced

½ cup (80 g) onion, chopped

1 cup (70 g) broccoli florets

8 ounces (225 g) mushrooms, sliced

1 cup (113 g) zucchini, sliced

1½ cups (355 ml) egg substitute

1 tablespoon (0.4 g) dried parsley

¼ teaspoon (0.5 g) black pepper

2 ounces (55 g) Swiss cheese, shredded

Spray a large oven-proof skillet with nonstick vegetable oil spray. Stir fry the red bell pepper, onions, and broccoli until crisp-tender. Add the mushrooms and zucchini and stir fry for 1 to 2 minutes more. Stir together the egg substitute, parsley, and pepper, and pour over vegetable mixture, spreading to cover. Cover and cook over medium heat for 10 to 12 minutes, or until eggs are nearly set. Sprinkle cheese over the top. Place under the broiler until eggs are set and cheese is melted.

—

Yield: 4 servings

PER SERVING: 140 calories (26% from fat, 51% from protein, 22% from carbohydrate); 18 g protein; 4 g total fat; 1 g saturated fat; 1 g monounsaturated fat; 2 g polyunsaturated fat; 8 g carbohydrate; 2 g fiber; 4 g sugar; 283 mg phosphorus; 209 mg calcium; 3 mg iron; 216 mg sodium; 721 mg potassium; 1618 IU vitamin A; 6 mg ATE vitamin E; 50 mg vitamin C; 6 mg cholesterol; 220 g water

Pasta Frittata

This makes a wonderful meatless meal. It's kind of like macaroni and cheese, only a little fancier.

2 tablespoons (30 ml) olive oil

1 cup (150 g) red bell pepper, diced

1 cup (160 g) onion, chopped

2 cups (100 g) cooked pasta

¼ cup (25 g) grated Parmesan

1 cup (235 ml) egg substitute

Heat a 10-inch (25-cm) nonstick skillet that is broiler safe. When the pan is hot, add the oil, then sauté red bell pepper and onion for 2 to 3 minutes, stirring frequently. Add the pasta to the pan, mixing well. When ingredients are thoroughly combined, press down on pasta with spatula to flatten it against the bottom of the pan. Let it cook a few minutes more. Whisk grated Parmesan into the egg substitute. Pour egg mixture over the top of the pasta, making sure the eggs spread evenly. Gently lift the edges of the pasta to let egg flow underneath and completely coat the pasta. Let the eggs cook for 6 to 9 minutes. Slide the pan into a preheated broiler and finish cooking.

—

Yield: 4 servings

PER SERVING: 360 calories (29% from fat, 20% from protein, 51% from carbohydrate); 18 g protein; 12 g total fat; 3 g saturated fat; 6 g monounsaturated fat; 2 g polyunsaturated fat; 46 g carbohydrate; 3 g fiber; 5 g sugar; 242 mg phosphorus; 125 mg calcium; 2 mg iron; 213 mg sodium; 469 mg potassium; 1421 IU vitamin A; 7 mg ATE vitamin E; 51 mg vitamin C; 6 mg cholesterol; 128 g water

Breakfast Cookies

These are good for breakfast on the run. They are fairly soft, but they're portable and fat-free.

3 cups (675 g) mashed banana

⅓ cup (82 g) applesauce

2 cups (160 g) quick-cooking oats

¼ cup (60 ml) skim milk

½ cup (75 g) dried cranberries

1 teaspoon (5 ml) vanilla

1 teaspoon (2.3 g) cinnamon

1 tablespoon (13 g) sugar

½ cup (50 g) pecans, chopped

Preheat oven to 350°F (180°C, or gas mark 4). Mix all ingredients in a bowl until well combined. Let this mixture stand for at least 5 minutes. Heap the dough by teaspoonfuls onto a greased baking sheet. Bake for 15 to 20 minutes and let cool.

—
Yield: 20 servings

PER SERVING: 127 calories (22% from fat, 10% from protein, 68% from carbohydrate); 3 g protein; 3 g total fat; 0 g saturated fat; 1 g monounsaturated fat; 1 g polyunsaturated fat; 23 g carbohydrate; 3 g fiber; 8 g sugar; 101 mg phosphorus; 18 mg calcium; 1 mg iron; 3 mg sodium; 209 mg potassium; 30 IU vitamin A; 2 mg ATE vitamin E; 3 mg vitamin C; 0 mg cholesterol; 33 g water

TIP

You can leave out the nuts if you prefer and substitute other dried fruit like raisins or dried apples for the cranberries.

Banana Melon Smoothies

I like smoothies for a quick breakfast, but I find that I'm often hungry before noon. Adding some extra protein with the tofu seems to help fill me up longer.

6 ounces (170 g) soft tofu

1 banana

1 cup (155 g) cantaloupe

½ cup (120 ml) skim milk

½ cup (120 ml) apple juice

Place all ingredients in a blender and process until smooth.

—
Yield: 2 servings

PER SERVING: 230 calories (11% from fat, 14% from protein, 75% from carbohydrate); 9 g protein; 3 g total fat; 1 g saturated fat; 1 g monounsaturated fat; 1 g polyunsaturated fat; 46 g carbohydrate; 4 g fiber; 28 g sugar; 164 mg phosphorus; 131 mg calcium; 1 mg iron; 60 mg sodium; 979 mg potassium; 3190 IU vitamin A; 38 mg ATE vitamin E; 43 mg vitamin C; 1 mg cholesterol; 347 g water

Bananaberry Smoothies

I developed this as a way to store and use later those last couple of bananas that always seem to be near the end of their useful life just when you don't have a use for them. Peel bananas, cut in halves or thirds, and freeze in a resealable plastic bag to use them in smoothies later. Using frozen bananas also gives you a nice, thick smoothie that isn't diluted by ice.

½ cup (120 ml) orange juice

1½ cups (340 g) frozen bananas

½ cup (55 g) frozen strawberries

Pour juice into blender. Add frozen bananas and berries and blend until smooth.

—

Yield: 2 servings

PER SERVING: 190 calories (4% from fat, 5% from protein, 91% from carbohydrate); 3 g protein; 1 g total fat; 0 g saturated fat; 0 g monounsaturated fat; 0 g polyunsaturated fat; 48 g carbohydrate; 5 g fiber; 22 g sugar; 53 mg phosphorus; 21 mg calcium; 1 mg iron; 3 mg sodium; 781 mg potassium; 161 IU vitamin A; 0 mg ATE vitamin E; 58 mg vitamin C; 0 mg cholesterol; 216 g water

TIP

You can use apple juice or other fruit juice and any kind of fresh or frozen fruit.

Peach Smoothies

The yogurt in this smoothie adds calcium, protein, and other nutrients, making it even more healthful than some of the fruit-only ones.

1 cup (235 ml) orange juice

1 cup (225 g) banana

1 cup (230 g) low fat vanilla yogurt

¾ cup (150 g) peaches, sliced and frozen

Place all ingredients in a blender and process until thick and smooth.

—
Yield: 1 serving

PER SERVING: 563 calories (7% from fat, 12% from protein, 81% from carbohydrate); 18 g protein; 5 g total fat; 2 g saturated fat; 1 g monounsaturated fat; 1 g polyunsaturated fat; 121 g carbohydrate; 8 g fiber; 71 g sugar; 431 mg phosphorus; 462 mg calcium; 1 mg iron; 166 mg sodium; 2034 mg potassium; 820 IU vitamin A; 29 mg ATE vitamin E; 111 mg vitamin C; 12 mg cholesterol; 685 g water

Strawberry Smoothie

1¼ cups (140 g) strawberries

1½ cups (355 ml) skim milk

1 tablespoon (13 g) sugar

1 teaspoon (5 ml) lemon juice

Put all ingredients in a blender and process until smooth.

—
Yield: 2 servings

PER SERVING: 131 calories (5% from fat, 24% from protein, 71% from carbohydrate); 8 g protein; 1 g total fat; 0 g saturated fat; 0 g monounsaturated fat; 0 g polyunsaturated fat; 24 g carbohydrate; 2 g fiber; 11 g sugar; 230 mg phosphorus; 279 mg calcium; 1 mg iron; 110 mg sodium; 484 mg potassium; 386 IU vitamin a; 113 mg ATE vitamin e; 59 mg vitamin c; 4 mg cholesterol; 254 g water

Yogurt Parfait

This makes a nice change of pace for breakfast. Even though the total fat may seem high, it's almost all from the walnuts, which provide a healthy fat.

1 cup (110 g) strawberries

2 tablespoons (26 g) sugar

8 ounces (225 g) plain fat-free yogurt

½ cup (50 g) granola

¼ cup (31 g) chopped walnuts

Chop the strawberries and toss with the sugar. Layer in parfait glasses in this order: fruit, yogurt, granola, and nuts. Repeat layers.

—

Yield: 2 servings

PER SERVING: 313 calories (29% from fat, 15% from protein, 55% from carbohydrate); 12 g protein; 11 g total fat; 1 g saturated fat; 3 g monounsaturated fat; 6 g polyunsaturated fat; 45 g carbohydrate; 4 g fiber; 32 g sugar; 333 mg phosphorus; 255 mg calcium; 1 mg iron; 166 mg sodium; 545 mg potassium; 23 IU vitamin A; 2 mg ATE vitamin E; 46 mg vitamin C; 2 mg cholesterol; 168 g water

3

Vegetable Mains

I have to admit that we never ate many vegetarian meals before my doctor warned me about my cholesterol. My wife sometimes claims to be a carnivore, and I have to admit to feeling that way myself sometimes. But as we learned to reduce the amount of saturated fats we were eating, we turned to vegetarian cooking more often. These recipes do contain cheese and other dairy products, so they wouldn't work without modification for vegan and other strict vegetarian diets. But for those of us looking for healthy alternatives to meat, they fill the bill.

Tomato and Basil Quiche

A great meatless quiche. If you want, you can put it in a crust, but we like it just as well without it.

1 tablespoon (15 ml) olive oil

1 cup (160 g) onion, sliced

2 cups (360 g) tomatoes, sliced

2 tablespoons (16 g) flour

2 teaspoons (1.4 g) dried basil

¾ cup (180 ml) egg substitute

½ cup (120 ml) skim milk

½ teaspoon (1 g) black pepper

1 cup (110 g) Swiss cheese, shredded

—
Yield: 4 servings

Preheat oven to 400°F (200°C, or gas mark 6). Heat olive oil in a large skillet over medium heat. Sauté onion until soft; remove from skillet. Sprinkle tomato slices with flour and basil, then sauté 1 minute on each side. In a small bowl, whisk together egg substitute and milk. Season with pepper. Spread half the cheese in the bottom of a pie pan sprayed with nonstick vegetable oil spray. Layer onions over the cheese and top with tomatoes. Pour the egg mixture over the vegetables. Sprinkle the remaining cheese over the top. Bake for 10 minutes. Reduce heat to 350°F (180°C, or gas mark 4), and bake for 15 to 20 minutes, or until filling is puffed and golden brown. Serve warm.

PER SERVING: 188 calories (33% from fat, 38% from protein, 29% from carbohydrate); 18 g protein; 7 g total fat; 2 g saturated fat; 3 g monounsaturated fat; 1 g polyunsaturated fat; 14 g carbohydrate; 2 g fiber; 2 g sugar; 327 mg phosphorus; 408 mg calcium; 2 mg iron; 196 mg sodium; 491 mg potassium; 781 IU vitamin A; 32 mg ATE vitamin E; 23 mg vitamin C; 13 mg cholesterol; 192 g water

Bean and Tomato Curry

This makes a good side dish with something like a grilled chicken breast or loin pork chop, but you can also use it for a vegetarian meal. In that case, serve over rice or with pita bread.

1 tablespoon (15 ml) canola oil

1 teaspoon (3.7 g) mustard seed

1 teaspoon (2.5 g) cumin seeds

1 cup (160 g) onion, chopped

1 tablespoon (6 g) fresh ginger, peeled and chopped

½ teaspoon (1.5 g) chopped garlic

4 cups (720 g) canned no-salt-added tomatoes

2 cups (450 g) kidney beans, drained and rinsed

1 teaspoon (2 g) curry powder

Heat oil in large pot over medium heat and stir-fry the mustard and cumin seeds until they pop. Add onion, ginger, and garlic, and stir-fry until lightly colored. Add tomatoes with juice, beans, and curry powder. Simmer for about 20 minutes or until thick and saucy.

—
Yield: 6 servings

PER SERVING: 140 calories (19% from fat, 19% from protein, 62% from carbohydrate); 7 g protein; 3 g total fat; 0 g saturated fat; 2 g monounsaturated fat; 1 g polyunsaturated fat; 23 g carbohydrate; 6 g fiber; 5 g sugar; 131 mg phosphorus; 81 mg calcium; 4 mg iron; 163 mg sodium; 598 mg potassium; 196 IU vitamin A; 0 mg ATE vitamin E; 18 mg vitamin C; 0 mg cholesterol; 215 g water

TIP

To lower the amount of sodium, use no-salt added beans or cooked dried beans.

Garbanzo Curry

Indian vegetarian slow cooker recipes like this curry will warm you up on a cold day. It's so easy, but it tastes as good as vegetarian Indian recipes you get at a restaurant.

2 tablespoons (30 ml) canola oil

1 cup (160 g) onion, diced

½ teaspoon (1.5 g) minced garlic

1 teaspoon (2.7 g) fresh ginger, peeled and grated

1 teaspoon (2.5 g) cumin

1 teaspoon (2 g) coriander

1 teaspoon (2.2 g) turmeric

2 cups (480 g) canned garbanzo beans, drained and rinsed

2 cups (360 g) canned no-salt-added tomatoes

½ teaspoon (1.2 g) garam masala

Heat oil in a heavy skillet. Sauté onion, garlic, ginger, cumin, coriander, and turmeric until onion becomes soft. Place onion mixture and remaining ingredients in a slow cooker and cook on low for 8 to 10 hours or on high for 4 to 5 hours.

—
Yield: 4 servings

PER SERVING: 246 calories (31% from fat, 12% from protein, 57% from carbohydrate); 8 g protein; 9 g total fat; 1 g saturated fat; 5 g monounsaturated fat; 3 g polyunsaturated fat; 37 g carbohydrate; 7 g fiber; 5 g sugar; 148 mg phosphorus; 93 mg calcium; 4 mg iron; 377 mg sodium; 524 mg potassium; 185 IU vitamin A; 0 mg ATE vitamin E; 20 mg vitamin C; 0 mg cholesterol; 233 g water

TIP

Garam masala is an Indian spice blend that you can find at larger grocery or specialty stores.

Tofu Curry

This is one of the simplest vegetarian meals you'll find. Serve the curry over rice with whatever condiments you like.

3 tablespoons (45 ml) olive oil, divided

12 ounces (340 g) firm tofu, drained and cubed

1 cup (113 g) zucchini, sliced

1 cup (70 g) mushrooms, sliced

1 cup (235 ml) fat-free evaporated milk

2 teaspoons (4 g) curry powder

Heat 1 tablespoon (15 ml) oil in a large skillet or work. Fry tofu until the bottom gets golden, then carefully turn and fry the other sides. Remove to a plate. Heat remaining oil and stir-fry zucchini and mushrooms until crisp-tender. Add milk and curry powder and continue cooking until slightly thickened. Stir in tofu.

—
Yield: 4 servings

PER SERVING: 204 calories (55% from fat, 23% from protein, 22% from carbohydrate); 12 g protein; 13 g total fat; 2 g saturated fat; 8 g monounsaturated fat; 2 g polyunsaturated fat; 12 g carbohydrate; 1 g fiber; 9 g sugar; 232 mg phosphorus; 223 mg calcium; 2 mg iron; 109 mg sodium; 531 mg potassium; 325 IU vitamin A; 76 mg ATE vitamin E; 7 mg vitamin C; 3 mg cholesterol; 171 g water

TIP

The possibilities for vegetable combinations are almost endless. Feel free to experiment.

Tofu and Broccoli Stir-Fry

This makes a quick and hearty meal with just rice as a base.

12 ounces (340 g) firm tofu

6 tablespoons (90 ml)
Reduced-Sodium Soy Sauce
(see recipe page 15)

2 tablespoons (30 ml) mirin wine

1 teaspoon (5 ml) sesame oil

¼ teaspoon (0.8 g) minced garlic

½ teaspoon (0.9 g) ground ginger

1 tablespoon (15 ml) olive oil

6 cups (420 g) broccoli florets

½ cup (35 g) mushrooms, sliced

Remove tofu from package and drain under a plate or other weight. Combine soy sauce, mirin, sesame oil, garlic, and ginger. Remove tofu from weight, cut into ¾-inch (2-cm) cubes, and place in soy sauce mixture. Heat olive oil in a wok or large skillet. Stir-fry broccoli and mushrooms until broccoli is crisp-tender. Remove from wok. Add tofu and cook until it begins to turn golden, then carefully turn and cook the other sides. Return vegetables to wok. Add remaining marinade. Cook and stir carefully until heated through.

—
Yield: 4 servings

PER SERVING: 155 calories (9% from fat, 5% from protein, 86% from carbohydrate); 9 g protein; 7 g total fat; 1 g saturated fat; 3 g monounsaturated fat; 5 g polyunsaturated fat; 156 g carbohydrate; 0 g fiber; 5 g sugar; 174 mg phosphorus; 92 mg calcium; 2 mg iron; 217 mg sodium; 606 mg potassium; 3204 IU vitamin A; 0 mg ATE vitamin E; 100 mg vitamin C; 0 mg cholesterol; 214 g water

Corn Chowder

This is great just the way it is, or you can add some cooked chicken or ground turkey if you like. We had it just like this with breadsticks and nothing else.

1 tablespoon (15 ml) olive oil

1 cup (160 g) onion, chopped

½ cup (50 g) celery, sliced

½ cup (65 g) carrot, sliced

2 tablespoons (16 g) flour

2 cups (475 ml) low sodium chicken broth

4 cups (945 ml) skim milk

2 potatoes, peeled and diced

3 cups (410 g) frozen corn, thawed

½ teaspoon (1 g) black pepper

Heat the oil in a large Dutch oven. Add the onion, celery, and carrots and cook over medium heat until just soft. Sprinkle on the flour and cook for 3 minutes, stirring frequently. Stir in the broth and milk. Add the potatoes and corn. Simmer for 25 minutes or until potatoes are tender. Sprinkle with pepper.

—
Yield: 6 servings

PER SERVING: 278 calories (12% from fat, 18% from protein, 70% from carbohydrate); 13 g protein; 4 g total fat; 1 g saturated fat; 2 g monounsaturated fat; 1 g polyunsaturated fat; 52 g carbohydrate; 5 g fiber; 6 g sugar; 346 mg phosphorus; 268 mg calcium; 2 mg iron; 148 mg sodium; 1148 mg potassium; 2176 IU vitamin A; 100 mg ATE vitamin E; 18 mg vitamin C; 3 mg cholesterol; 427 g water

Vegetarian Chili

This is a different kind of chili, but it's still very good. Garnish with fresh cilantro, crushed corn chips, shredded low fat cheese, or fat-free sour cream (or all of them!).

¼ cup (60 ml) dry sherry

1 tablespoon (15 ml) olive oil

2 cups (320 g) onion, chopped

½ cup (50 g) celery, chopped

½ cup (65 g) carrot, sliced

½ cup (75 g) red bell pepper, chopped

4 cups (900 g) cooked black beans

2 cups (475 ml) water

½ teaspoon (1.5 g) minced garlic

1 cup (180 g) plum tomato, chopped

2 teaspoons (5 g) ground cumin

4 teaspoons (10 g) chili powder

½ teaspoon (0.5 g) dried oregano

¼ cup (15 g) chopped fresh cilantro

2 tablespoons (30 ml) honey

2 tablespoons (30 ml) no-salt-added tomato paste

In a large, heavy pot over medium heat, combine sherry and oil and heat to simmering. Add onions and sauté 8 to 10 minutes. Add celery, carrots, and bell pepper and sauté 5 minutes more, stirring frequently. Add remaining ingredients and bring to a boil. Lower heat and simmer, covered, for 45 minutes to 1 hour. Mixture should be thick, with all water absorbed.

—
Yield: 8 servings

PER SERVING: 192 calories (12% from fat, 18% from protein, 69% from carbohydrate); 9 g protein; 3 g total fat; 0 g saturated fat; 1 g monounsaturated fat; 1 g polyunsaturated fat; 34 g carbohydrate; 10 g fiber; 9 g sugar; 155 mg phosphorus; 55 mg calcium; 3 mg iron; 35 mg sodium; 563 mg potassium; 2358 IU vitamin A; 0 mg ATE vitamin E; 20 mg vitamin C; 0 mg cholesterol; 201 g water

Grilled Veggie Subs

I particularly like these on focaccia bread, but they are also good on homemade rolls. You could add a slice of chicken or other leftover meat if you aren't into the all-veggie thing, but I don't see the need. Feel free to vary the vegetables as desired. I usually sprinkle a little homemade Italian dressing on them too.

4 slices red onion

½ cup (35 g) mushrooms, sliced

½ cup (56 g) zucchini, sliced

¾ cup (112 g) eggplant, sliced

1 cup (180 g) tomato, sliced

2 tablespoons (30 ml) olive oil

8 ounces (225 g) Swiss cheese, sliced

8 slices focaccia bread or 4 rolls

Preheat broiler. Brush onion, mushrooms, zucchini, eggplant, and tomato with oil. Grill or sauté until soft. Divide evenly between focaccia or rolls. Top each with a slice of Swiss cheese. Place under the broiler until cheese melts.

—
Yield: 4 servings

PER SERVING: 192 calories (46% from fat, 36% from protein, 18% from carbohydrate); 17 g protein; 10 g total fat; 3 g saturated fat; 6 g monounsaturated fat; 1 g polyunsaturated fat; 9 g carbohydrate; 2 g fiber; 4 g sugar; 381 mg phosphorus; 562 mg calcium; 0 mg iron; 153 mg sodium; 313 mg potassium; 432 IU vitamin A; 22 mg ATE vitamin E; 11 mg vitamin C; 20 mg cholesterol; 142 g water

TIP

Be prepared with extra napkins—these are very juicy!

Grilled Stuffed Portobellos

I discovered Portobello mushrooms not too long ago. We like them grilled on a bun, but these Mediterranean-flavored ones are better served with pasta or rice.

⅔ cup (120 g) plum tomato, chopped

2 ounces (55 g) part-skim mozzarella, shredded

1 teaspoon (5 ml) olive oil, divided

½ teaspoon (0.4 g) fresh rosemary

⅛ teaspoon (0.3 g) coarsely ground black pepper

¼ teaspoon (0.8 g) crushed garlic

4 Portobello mushroom caps, about 4 to 5 inches (10 to 12.5 cm) each

2 tablespoons (30 ml) lemon juice

2 teaspoons (2.6 g) fresh parsley

Prepare grill. Combine the tomato, cheese, ½ teaspoon (2.5 ml) oil, rosemary, pepper, and garlic in a small bowl. Remove brown gills from the undersides of mushroom caps using a spoon, and discard gills. Remove stems; discard. Combine remaining ½ teaspoon oil (2.5 ml) and lemon juice in a small bowl. Brush over both sides of mushroom caps. Place the mushroom caps, stem sides down, on grill rack sprayed with nonstick vegetable oil spray, and grill for 5 minutes on each side or until soft. Spoon one-quarter of the tomato mixture into each mushroom cap. Cover and grill 3 minutes or until cheese is melted. Sprinkle with parsley.

—
Yield: 4 servings

PER SERVING: 75 calories (40% from fat, 29% from protein, 32% from carbohydrate); 6 g protein; 4 g total fat; 2 g saturated fat; 1 g monounsaturated fat; 0 g polyunsaturated fat; 6 g carbohydrate; 2 g fiber; 3 g sugar; 181 mg phosphorus; 122 mg calcium; 1 mg iron; 95 mg sodium; 490 mg potassium; 331 IU vitamin A; 18 mg ATE vitamin E; 8 mg vitamin C; 9 mg cholesterol; 115 g water

Zucchini Wraps

A nice change-of-pace zucchini dish, vegetarian and flavored with southwestern spices.

1 tablespoon (15 ml) olive oil

1 cup (160 g) onion, chopped

1 teaspoon (3 g) dry mustard

1 teaspoon (2.5 g) cumin

4 cups (500 g) zucchini, shredded

½ teaspoon (1.3 g) chili powder

¼ teaspoon (0.5 g) black pepper

4 tortillas

¼ cup (60 g) fat-free sour cream

In a medium wok or frying pan, heat the oil over medium-high heat. Add the onions, mustard, and cumin. Sauté until onions are soft. Add the shredded zucchini. Cook 5 to 10 minutes, stirring frequently, until the zucchini gets soft and tender. Stir in the chili powder and pepper. Warm the tortillas and place on a flat surface. Spread 1 tablespoon (15 g) of sour cream on each. Place one-quarter of the zucchini filling in the center of each tortilla. Roll up each tortilla.

—
Yield: 4 servings

PER SERVING: 131 calories (32% from fat, 12% from protein, 56% from carbohydrate); 4 g protein; 4 g total fat; 1 g saturated fat; 3 g monounsaturated fat; 1 g polyunsaturated fat; 17 g carbohydrate; 3 g fiber; 4 g sugar; 135 mg phosphorus; 66 mg calcium; mg iron; 33 mg sodium; 456 mg potassium; 406 IU vitamin A; 15 mg ATE vitamin E; 24 mg vitamin C; 6 mg cholesterol; 174 g water

Whole Wheat Apple Strata

This has become a traditional Christmas-morning breakfast. The original recipe called for ham, but no one seems to miss it. You could use any leftover bread, but I like honey wheat. If you can't find canned apples, you can use apple pie filling, although the result will be sweeter.

6 slices whole wheat bread, cubed

1 can (21-ounce, or 600 g) apples or apple pie filling

3 ounces (85 g) low fat cheddar cheese, shredded

1 cup (235 ml) egg substitute

¼ cup (60 ml) skim milk

Place bread in a 9-inch (23-cm) square pan coated with nonstick vegetable oil spray. Spoon apples over bread. Sprinkle with cheese. Combine egg substitute and milk and pour over bread mixture. Cover with plastic wrap and refrigerate overnight. Preheat oven to 350°F (180°C, or gas mark 4). Bake uncovered for 40 to 45 minutes, or until top is lightly browned and center is set.

—
Yield: 4 servings

PER SERVING: 232 calories (21% from fat, 31% from protein, 48% from carbohydrate); 18 g protein; 5 g total fat; 2 g saturated fat; 2 g monounsaturated fat; 2 g polyunsaturated fat; 28 g carbohydrate; 3 g fiber; 9 g sugar; 284 mg phosphorus; 189 mg calcium; 3 mg iron; 484 mg sodium; 376 mg potassium; 313 IU vitamin A; 22 mg ATE vitamin E; 2 mg vitamin C; 5 mg cholesterol; 125 g water

4

Fish Mains

We already talked about fish and identified it as a major source of omega-3 fatty acids, which are helpful in reducing LDL cholesterol levels. That's the good news. The really good news is that fish comes in a variety of flavors, which makes it great as a stand-alone dish as well as being ideal for any number of recipes with herbs or sauces and in soups and stews. This chapter contains a wide range of recipes, so eating your two servings a week should not be a problem.

Baked Swordfish with Vegetables

This is a fairly simple recipe, with the flavor coming from the vegetables. It's good with pasta or plain brown rice.

4 ounces (115 g) mushrooms, sliced

1 cup (160 g) onion, sliced

2 tablespoons (19 g) green bell pepper, chopped

2 tablespoons (30 ml) lemon juice

¼ teaspoon (0.3 g) dried dill

1 pound (455 g) swordfish steaks

4 small bay leaves

2 tomatoes, sliced

Preheat oven to 400°F (200°C, or gas mark 6). In a bowl, combine mushrooms, onions, green bell pepper, lemon juice, and dill. Line a shallow baking pan with foil. Spread vegetable mixture in bottom then arrange swordfish steaks on top. Place a bay leaf on each swordfish steak. Place 2 tomato slices on each swordfish steak. Cover pan with foil and bake for 45 to 55 minutes or until fish flakes easily with a fork.

—
Yield: 4 servings

PER SERVING: 165 calories (26% from fat, 59% from protein, 15% from carbohydrate); 24 g protein; 5 g total fat; 1 g saturated fat; 2 g monounsaturated fat; 1 g polyunsaturated fat; 6 g carbohydrate; 1 g fiber; 3 g sugar; 339 mg phosphorus; 18 mg calcium; 1 mg iron; 126 mg sodium; 529 mg potassium; 168 IU vitamin A; 41 mg ATE vitamin E; 12 mg vitamin C; 44 mg cholesterol; 159 g water

Creole-Style Catfish

A simple, Creole-style recipe.

1 tablespoon (15 ml) olive oil

1 cup (160 g) onion, chopped

½ cup (50 g) celery, chopped

½ cup (75 g) green bell pepper, chopped

1 clove garlic, minced

2 cups (360 g) canned no-salt-added tomatoes

1 lemon, sliced

1 tablespoon (15 ml) Worcestershire sauce

1 tablespoon (7 g) paprika

1 bay leaf

¼ teaspoon (0.3 g) dried thyme

¼ teaspoon (1 ml) hot pepper sauce

2 pounds (905 g) catfish fillets

Heat the oil in a large skillet over medium heat. Add the onion, celery, green pepper, and garlic. Cook until soft. Add tomatoes and their liquid. Break the tomatoes with a spoon. Add lemon slices, Worcestershire sauce, paprika, bay leaf, thyme, and hot pepper sauce. Cook, stirring occasionally, for 15 minutes, or until the sauce is slightly thickened. Press fish pieces down into sauce and spoon some of the sauce over the top of the fish. Cover the pan and simmer gently for 10 minutes, or until the fish flakes easily with a fork. Serve over hot cooked rice.

Yield: 6 servings

PER SERVING: 260 calories (49% from fat, 38% from protein, 13% from carbohydrate); 25 g protein; 14 g total fat; 3 g saturated fat; 7 g monounsaturated fat; 3 g polyunsaturated fat; 9 g carbohydrate; 2 g fiber; 4 g sugar; 341 mg phosphorus; 55 mg calcium; 2 mg iron; 125 mg sodium; 746 mg potassium; 870 IU vitamin A; 23 mg ATE vitamin E; 31 mg vitamin C; 71 mg cholesterol; 242 g water

TIP

You can substitute any other white fish for the catfish.

Herbed Fish

Simple baked fish made flavorful by a combination of herbs and spices.

2 pounds (905 g) perch, or other firm white fish

1 tablespoon (15 ml) olive oil

½ teaspoon (1.5 g) garlic powder

½ teaspoon (0.3 g) dried marjoram

½ teaspoon (0.5 g) dried thyme

⅛ teaspoon (0.3 g) white pepper

2 bay leaves

½ cup (80 g) onion, chopped

½ cup (120 ml) white wine

Preheat oven to 350°F (180°C, or gas mark 4). Wash fish, pat dry, and place in 9 × 13-inch (23 × 33-cm) dish. Combine oil with garlic powder, marjoram, thyme, and white pepper. Drizzle over fish. Top with bay leaves and onion. Pour wine over all. Bake, uncovered, for 20 to 30 minutes, or until fish flakes easily with a fork.

—

Yield: 4 servings

PER SERVING: 277 calories (26% from fat, 69% from protein, 5% from carbohydrate); 43 g protein; 7 g total fat; 1 g saturated fat; 4 g monounsaturated fat; 1 g polyunsaturated fat; 3 g carbohydrate; 0 g fiber; 1 g sugar; 503 mg phosphorus; 253 mg calcium; 2 mg iron; 173 mg sodium; 675 mg potassium; 100 IU vitamin A; 27 mg ATE vitamin E; 3 mg vitamin C; 95 mg cholesterol; 222 g water

Spaghetti with Fish

My daughter made this after seeing a similar recipe on some cooking program on TV. It turned out really well and is just different enough from the way we typically serve pasta that we tend to go back to it when we want something a little different, especially since it fits my daughter's rule that if you don't know what to have, make something Italian.

8 ounces (225 g) spaghetti

1 pound (455 g) perch, or other white fish

2 tablespoons (30 ml) olive oil

½ teaspoon (1.5 g) minced garlic

2 tablespoons (30 ml) lemon juice

1 tablespoon (2.5 g) Italian seasoning

¼ teaspoon (0.5 g) black pepper

2 cups (360 g) canned no-salt-added tomatoes

¼ cup (60 ml) white wine

2 tablespoons (8 g) fresh parsley

Cook spaghetti according to package directions, drain and set aside. Cut fish into 1-inch (2.5-cm) cubes. In a large skillet heat olive oil. Add garlic, lemon juice, Italian seasoning, and pepper. Cook until garlic starts to brown. Add fish and cook until nearly done. Add tomatoes and reheat to boiling. Remove from heat. Stir in spaghetti and wine and toss to coat spaghetti with sauce. Sprinkle with parsley.

—

Yield: 4 servings

PER SERVING: 276 calories (31% from fat, 35% from protein, 34% from carbohydrate); 24 g protein; 9 g total fat; 1 g saturated fat; 6 g monounsaturated fat; 1 g polyunsaturated fat; 22 g carbohydrate; 4 g fiber; 3 g sugar; 317 mg phosphorus; 177 mg calcium; 3 mg iron; 103 mg sodium; 599 mg potassium; 430 IU vitamin A; 14 mg ATE vitamin E; 19 mg vitamin C; 48 mg cholesterol; 263 g water

Fish Sauce for Pasta

Even though this recipe may seem higher in fat than most of the others, it's the good kind of fat that comes from olive oil and fish. So enjoy it guilt-free.

¼ cup (60 ml) olive oil

12 ounces (340 g) salmon fillets, cubed

12 ounces (340 g) cod fillets, cubed

1 teaspoon (3 g) minced garlic

½ cup (120 ml) white wine

½ teaspoon (0.5 g) dried oregano

½ teaspoon (0.6 g) dried rosemary

1 teaspoon (0.1 g) dried parsley

1 tablespoon (10 g) onion, minced

Heat oil in a heavy skillet. Add salmon, cod, and garlic and sauté for a minute or two, until nearly cooked through. Add wine and remaining ingredients and continue cooking until sauce has been reduced to about half. Serve over pasta.

—
Yield: 6 servings

PER SERVING: 248 calories (61% from fat, 37% from protein, 2% from carbohydrate); 21 g protein; 16 g total fat; 3 g saturated fat; 9 g monounsaturated fat; 3 g polyunsaturated fat; 1 g carbohydrate; 0 g fiber; 0 g sugar; 252 mg phosphorus; 21 mg calcium; 1 mg iron; 66 mg sodium; 461 mg potassium; 76 IU vitamin A; 15 mg ATE vitamin E; 3 mg vitamin C; 58 mg cholesterol; 104 g water

Tuna Noodle Casserole

This is traditional American comfort food.

1 tablespoon (15 ml) olive oil

2 tablespoons (16 g) flour

2 cups (470 ml) skim milk

¼ cup (30 g) low fat cheddar
cheese, shredded

3 cups (450 g) cooked egg noodles

10-ounce (280 g) package
frozen peas, thawed

7 ounces (200 g) water-packed tuna

4 ounces (115 g) mushrooms, sliced

¼ cup (37 g) chopped green
bell pepper

⅛ teaspoon (0.3 g) black pepper

½ cup (60 g) bread crumbs

Preheat oven to 375°F (190°C, or gas mark 5). Heat oil in a large skillet over low heat; add flour, stirring until smooth. Cook 1 minute, stirring constantly. Gradually add milk; cook over medium heat, stirring constantly, until mixture is thickened and bubbly. Stir in cheese; cook over low heat, stirring constantly, until cheese melts. Remove from heat. Combine cheese sauce, noodles, and next 5 ingredients (through black pepper). Spoon mixture into a 2-quart (1.9-L) casserole dish coated with nonstick vegetable oil spray. Sprinkle evenly with bread crumbs. Bake for 35 minutes, or until the casserole is bubbly and the top is browned.

—
Yield: 6 servings

PER SERVING: 277 calories (14% from fat, 28% from protein, 58% from carbohydrate); 19 g protein; 4 g total fat; 1 g saturated fat; 2 g monounsaturated fat; 1 g polyunsaturated fat; 40 g carbohydrate; 7 g fiber; 3 g sugar; 303 mg phosphorus; 174 mg calcium; 2 mg iron; 414 mg sodium; 424 mg potassium; 1254 IU vitamin A; 59 mg ATE vitamin E; 11 mg vitamin C; 13 mg cholesterol; 211 g water

Swedish Salmon Stew

This recipe turned up one night during a fairly desperate search for something different to do with fish.

1½ **pounds (680 g) potatoes, peeled and sliced**

1½ **pounds (680 g) salmon fillets**

1 **tablespoon (4 g) fresh dill, chopped**

¼ **cup (60 ml) olive oil, heated**

½ **cup (120 ml) white wine**

¼ **cup (60 ml) sherry**

½ **cup (115 g) fat-free sour cream**

2 **tablespoons (30 g) horseradish, grated**

Preheat oven to 350°F (180°C, or gas mark 4). Boil potatoes for 10 to 15 minutes, or until almost done. Layer potato slices in a large ovenproof casserole. Place the salmon on top. Sprinkle with the dill and drizzle with the olive oil. Cover and bake for 25 minutes. Remove from the oven and pour the wine and sherry over. Continue to cook uncovered until salmon flakes easily with a fork. Stir together sour cream and horseradish and pour over the top.

—
Yield: 6 servings

PER SERVING: 372 calories (50% from fat, 24% from protein, 26% from carbohydrate); 19 g protein; 18 g total fat; 3 g saturated fat; 6 g monounsaturated fat; 8 g polyunsaturated fat; 22 g carbohydrate; 2 g fiber; 3 g sugar; 288 mg phosphorus; 57 mg calcium; 1 mg iron; 82 mg sodium; 891 mg potassium; 154 IU vitamin A; 32 mg ATE vitamin E; 15 mg vitamin C; 56 mg cholesterol; 193 g water

Greek Fish Stew

This is a soup to warm you on a cold night. A slice of bread is all that's needed to make it a meal.

4 ounces (115 g) orzo, or other
small pasta

½ cup (80 g) onion, chopped

½ teaspoon (1.5 g) minced garlic

1 teaspoon (2 g) fennel seed

2 cups (360 g) canned no-salt-added
tomatoes

2 cups (470 g) low sodium
chicken broth

1 tablespoon (0.4 g) dried parsley

½ teaspoon (1 g) black pepper

¼ teaspoon (0.6 g) turmeric

12 ounces (340 g) cod fillets,
cut in 1-inch (2.5-cm) cubes

Cook pasta according to package directions. Drain and set aside. In a large nonstick saucepan coated with nonstick vegetable oil spray, cook onions, garlic, and fennel seed until onion is tender. Add tomatoes, broth, parsley, pepper, and turmeric. Reduce heat and simmer for 10 minutes. Add fish and simmer for 5 minutes, or until fish is cooked through. Divide pasta among four bowls. Ladle soup over pasta.

—

Yield: 4 servings

PER SERVING: 226 calories (8% from fat, 40% from protein, 53% from carbohydrate); 23 g protein; 2 g total fat; 0 g saturated fat; 1 g monounsaturated fat; 1 g polyunsaturated fat; 30 g carbohydrate; 3 g fiber; 5 g sugar; 295 mg phosphorus; 75 mg calcium; 3 mg iron; 101 mg sodium; 794 mg potassium; 255 IU vitamin A; 10 mg ATE vitamin E; 15 mg vitamin C; 37 mg cholesterol; 319 g water

Fish Wine Chowder

My daughter fixed this one rainy cold night. Since she isn't a fish lover, I figured it must be the amount of wine in it that appealed to her. It turns out to be a liberal modification of a recipe in a *Better Homes and Gardens* soup cookbook. It turned out quite well, and even she had to admit that fish isn't bad this way. You could use whatever fish you have on hand or that you prefer; the salmon and perch just happened to be what was in our freezer.

1 pound (455 g) salmon

1 pound (455 g) perch

4 slices low sodium bacon

½ cup (80 g) onion, chopped

½ cup (50 g) celery, chopped

¼ teaspoon (0.8 g) minced garlic

1½ cups (355 ml) white wine

1½ cups (355 ml) water

2 potatoes, cubed

¼ teaspoon (0.3 g) thyme

1 teaspoon (0.1 g) parsley

3 tablespoons (24 g) flour

3 tablespoons (45 ml) water

½ cup (60 ml) skim milk

Cut fish into cubes; set aside. Cook bacon in a Dutch oven; crumble and set aside. Drain grease from pan. Sauté onion, celery, and garlic until tender. Add wine, water, potatoes, thyme, and parsley. Simmer for 20 minutes, or until potatoes are almost done. Add fish, cover and simmer 10 minutes more. Mix together flour and water to form a paste. Stir into soup and simmer until thickened. Stir in milk and reserved bacon.

—
Yield: 8 servings

PER SERVING: 306 calories (30% from fat, 39% from protein, 31% from carbohydrate); 26 g protein; 9 g total fat; 2 g saturated fat; 3 g monounsaturated fat; 3 g polyunsaturated fat; 21 g carbohydrate; 2 g fiber; 2 g sugar; 368 mg phosphorus; 113 mg calcium; 2 mg iron; 142 mg sodium; 913 mg potassium; 133 IU vitamin A; 25 mg ATE vitamin E; 13 mg vitamin C; 62 mg cholesterol; 285 g water

Tuna Chowder

We like this for dinner with some freshly baked bread. It makes a nice warm meal on a cool evening, and it's the kind of thing you can throw together quickly when you haven't planned something for dinner.

2 cups (470 ml) water

2 cups (470 ml) low sodium chicken broth

6 potatoes, diced

14 ounces (400 g) water-packed tuna

½ cup (65 g) carrots, sliced

½ cup (50 g) celery, sliced

½ cup (80 g) onion, diced

½ cup (82 g) frozen corn, thawed

½ teaspoon (0.3 g) dried basil

½ teaspoon (0.5 g) dried dill

1 tablespoon (0.4 g) dried parsley

½ cup (120 ml) skim milk

In a large saucepan, mix water with broth. Add potatoes and simmer for 10 to 15 minutes, or until tender. Remove cooked potatoes from broth, reserving liquid. Purée cooked potatoes with ¼ cup (60 ml) reserved broth. Add tuna, carrots, celery, onion, corn, basil, dill, parsley, and puréed potatoes to remaining broth in saucepan. Simmer for 8 to 10 minutes, or until vegetables are tender. Stir in milk and heat to serving temperature, but do not boil.

—
Yield: 6 servings

PER SERVING: 379 calories (4% from fat, 28% from protein, 68% from carbohydrate); 27 g protein; 2 g total fat; 0 g saturated fat; 0 g monounsaturated fat; 1 g polyunsaturated fat; 66 g carbohydrate; 7 g fiber; 5 g sugar; 398 mg phosphorus; 93 mg calcium; 4 mg iron; 300 mg sodium; 2047 mg potassium; 2000 IU vitamin A; 24 mg ATE vitamin E; 35 mg vitamin C; 20 mg cholesterol; 562 g water

Oven-Steamed Salmon and Vegetables

I've also cooked this on a gas grill.

8 ounces (225 g) salmon fillets

2 medium potatoes, diced

½ cup (56 g) yellow squash, thinly sliced

½ cup (65 g) carrot, thinly sliced

¼ cup (25 g) scallions, thinly sliced

½ cup (35 g) mushrooms, sliced

2 teaspoons (10 ml) white wine

½ teaspoon (0.5 g) dried dill

½ teaspoon (1.5 g) minced garlic

¼ teaspoon (0.5 g) black pepper, fresh ground

Preheat oven to 425°F (220°C, or gas mark 7). Place a baking sheet in the oven to preheat as well. Meanwhile, spray the center of two 12-inch (30-cm) squares of aluminum foil with nonstick vegetable oil spray. Combine salmon, potatoes, squash, carrots, scallions, and mushrooms and divide evenly among the prepared foil sheets. Sprinkle with wine, dill, garlic, and pepper; fold diagonally to form a triangle; tightly seal edges. Place foil package on preheated baking sheet, then return to oven and bake 10 to 15 minutes, or until salmon is opaque and vegetables are tender.

—
Yield: 2 servings

PER SERVING: 498 calories (23% from fat, 25% from protein, 52% from carbohydrate); 31 g protein; 13 g total fat; 3 g saturated fat; 4 g monounsaturated fat; 5 g polyunsaturated fat; 65 g carbohydrate; 8 g fiber; 6 g sugar; 535 mg phosphorus; 82 mg calcium; 4 mg iron; 116 mg sodium; 2374 mg potassium; 5659 IU vitamin A; 17 mg ATE vitamin E; 46 mg vitamin C; 67 mg cholesterol; 464 g water

5

Poultry Mains

Chicken and turkey are great choices for a low cholesterol diet. You can hardly find any other meat with lower saturated fat than chicken or turkey breast. And the rest of the birds are healthy too, as long as you avoid eating the skin. There are a lot of chicken breast recipes here because they are a staple of a low fat diet. The only potential problem with chicken breasts is they can be dry and tough if you aren't careful cooking them. Many of these recipes contain sauces and marinades that help to keep them moist and give them extra flavor. There also are healthy recipes here for whole birds and ground turkey, so you don't need to worry about variety. I've even included some recipes that give you the taste of fried chicken, while still holding the line on fat.

Baked Italian Chicken Breasts

This is really "oven-fried" chicken. Using boneless breasts cuts way back on the saturated fat. And the sun-dried tomatoes and Italian seasoning give it a different flavor. We had this recently with roasted vegetables that we also sprinkled with Italian seasoning.

2 boneless chicken breasts

½ cup (60 g) bread crumbs

¼ cup (28 g) oil-packed
sun-dried tomatoes

¼ teaspoon (0.8 g) garlic powder

1 teaspoon (0.7 g) Italian seasoning

¼ cup (60 ml) egg substitute

Preheat oven to 400°F (200°C, or gas mark 6). Split each chicken breast in half to make two thin cutlets. Combine bread crumbs, tomatoes, garlic powder, and Italian seasoning in a food processor. Process until well blended. Dip chicken in egg substitute and then in crumb mixture to coat thoroughly. Place in an ovenproof casserole dish. Bake for 20 minutes, or until chicken is cooked through.

—
Yield: 2 servings

PER SERVING: 243 calories (20% from fat, 41% from protein, 39% from carbohydrate); 25 g protein; 5 g total fat; 1 g saturated fat; 2 g monounsaturated fat; 2 g polyunsaturated fat; 23 g carbohydrate; 2 g fiber; 2 g sugar; 243 mg phosphorus; 88 mg calcium; 3 mg iron; 336 mg sodium; 565 mg potassium; 339 IU vitamin A; 4 mg ATE vitamin E; 15 mg vitamin C; 41 mg cholesterol; 88 g water

Chicken with Red Pepper Sauce

This was a recipe that sat in my "I need to try that" file for a while. It had a great flavor, but wasn't overly hot.

FOR CHICKEN:

¼ cup (30 g) flour

½ teaspoon (1.3 g) paprika

¼ teaspoon (0.5 g) black pepper

2 pounds (905 g) boneless chicken breasts

FOR SAUCE:

1 tablespoon (15 ml) canola oil

¾ cup (113 g) red bell pepper, cut in 1-inch (2.5-cm) cubes

¼ cup (25 g) scallions, sliced

2 tablespoons (16 g) flour

1 cup (235 ml) low sodium chicken broth

2 tablespoons (26 g) sugar

½ tablespoon (2.5 g) cayenne pepper

⅓ cup (80 ml) cider vinegar

Preheat oven to 375°F (190°C, or gas mark 5).

TO MAKE THE CHICKEN: In a plastic bag, combine flour, paprika, and pepper. Add chicken, a few pieces at a time, to the bag, shaking to coat well. Arrange chicken in a shallow baking pan. Coat with nonstick vegetable oil spray to moisten the flour. Bake for 20 minutes.

TO MAKE THE SAUCE: Heat the oil in a medium saucepan; cook red bell pepper and scallions until tender. Stir in flour. Add chicken broth, sugar, and cayenne pepper. Cook and stir until thickened and bubbly. Cook and stir for 1 minute more. Remove from heat, stir in vinegar, and cool slightly. Spoon sauce over chicken. Bake for 20 minutes more, or until done, basting with the sauce 2 or 3 times during baking.

—

Yield: 6 servings

PER SERVING: 249 calories (18% from fat, 61% from protein, 21% from carbohydrate); 37 g protein; 5 g total fat; 1 g saturated fat; 2 g monounsaturated fat; 1 g polyunsaturated fat; 13 g carbohydrate; 1 g fiber; 5 g sugar; 326 mg phosphorus; 26 mg calcium; 2 mg iron; 113 mg sodium; 503 mg potassium; 942 IU vitamin A; 9 mg ATE vitamin E; 27 mg vitamin C; 88 mg cholesterol; 186 g water

TIP

If you want something a little spicier, just increase the amount of cayenne pepper.

Indian Chicken

A slightly tangy, not overly hot chicken flavored like the classic Tandoori chicken. If you like hotter food, you can add more cayenne pepper.

1 cup (230 g) plain fat-free yogurt

½ teaspoon (0.9 g) cardamom

½ teaspoon (1.3 g) ground cumin

½ teaspoon (1.1 g) turmeric

⅛ teaspoon (0.3 g) cayenne pepper

1 teaspoon (0.6 g) bay leaf, crushed

½ teaspoon (1.5 g) garlic powder

¾ teaspoon (1.4 g) ground ginger

¼ cup (40 g) onion, minced

¼ cup (60 ml) lime juice

¼ teaspoon (0.5 g) black pepper

1 teaspoon (2.3 g) cinnamon

1 teaspoon (2 g) ground coriander

8 boneless chicken breasts

Combine yogurt and remaining ingredients except chicken, mixing well. Prick chicken with a fork. In a resealable plastic bag or glass pan large enough to hold chicken, cover chicken with yogurt marinade, making sure all surfaces of chicken are coated. Cover and refrigerate at least 3 hours, or overnight. Turn at least once while marinating. Grill over medium heat until done or preheat oven to 375°F (190°C, or gas mark 5) and place chicken in a greased roasting pan with marinade and cook for 45 minutes to 1 hour, or until chicken is tender.

—
Yield: 8 servings

PER SERVING: 103 calories (9% from fat, 73% from protein, 17% from carbohydrate); 18 g protein; 1 g total fat; 0 g saturated fat; 0 g monounsaturated fat; 0 g polyunsaturated fat; 4 g carbohydrate; 0 g fiber; 3 g sugar; 193 mg phosphorus; 79 mg calcium; 1 mg iron; 71 mg sodium; 293 mg potassium; 44 IU vitamin A; 5 mg ATE vitamin E; 4 mg vitamin C; 42 mg cholesterol; 91 g water

Reduced-Fat Chicken and Dumplings

This is classic comfort food any time of year, but especially as the weather gets colder. You can also make the dumplings using 2 cups (250 g) of Reduced-Fat Biscuit Mix (see recipe page 19) rather than the flour, baking powder, and margarine called for here.

FOR CHICKEN:

1½ cups (165 g) chicken breast, cooked and cubed

3 cups (710 ml) low sodium chicken broth

3 cups (710 ml) water

1½ cups (195 g) carrot, sliced

6 potatoes, peeled and cubed

1 cup (160 g) onion, chopped

FOR DUMPLINGS:

2 cups (250 g) flour

1 tablespoon (14 g) baking powder

2 tablespoons (28 g) margarine

⅔ cup (160 g) skim milk

TO MAKE THE CHICKEN: Place chicken, broth, water, carrots, potatoes, and onion in a large pan. Bring to a boil.

TO MAKE THE DUMPLINGS: Stir together the flour and baking powder. Cut in margarine until mixture resembles coarse crumbs. Stir in milk until dough holds together in a ball. Drop dumplings on top of boiling chicken mixture by spoonfuls. Reduce heat and simmer uncovered for 10 minutes. Cover and simmer 10 minutes more.

—
Yield: 6 servings

PER SERVING: 556 calories (11% from fat, 19% from protein, 71% from carbohydrate); 26 g protein; 7 g total fat; 2 g saturated fat; 3 g monounsaturated fat; 1 g polyunsaturated fat; 100 g carbohydrate; 9 g fiber; 7 g sugar; 488 mg phosphorus; 251 mg calcium; 6 mg iron; 413 mg sodium; 2113 mg potassium; 5668 IU vitamin A; 65 mg ATE vitamin E; 36 mg vitamin C; 30 mg cholesterol; 637 g water

Chicken and Spaghetti Bake

This comes more or less directly from my daughter's theory of cooking, namely, if you can't think of anything else for dinner, make something Italian. Works for me!

8 ounces (225 g) spaghetti

½ cup (120 ml) egg substitute

1 cup (225 g) fat-free cottage cheese

1 pound (455 g) boneless chicken breast, sliced

½ cup (80 g) onion, chopped

½ cup (75 g) green bell pepper, chopped

2 cups (360 g) canned no-salt-added tomatoes

6 ounces (170 g) no-salt-added tomato paste

1 teaspoon (4 g) sugar

1 teaspoon (1 g) dried oregano

½ teaspoon (1.5 g) garlic powder

½ cup (60 g) mozzarella, shredded

Preheat oven to 350°F (180°C, or gas mark 4). Cook spaghetti according to package directions. Drain. Mix in egg substitute. Form into a "crust" in a greased 10-inch (25-cm) pie pan. Top with cottage cheese. In a large skillet cook chicken, onion, and green bell pepper until meat is done and vegetables are tender. Add remaining ingredients except mozzarella and heat through. Spread over spaghetti and cottage cheese. Bake for 20 minutes. Sprinkle with mozzarella about 5 minutes before the end of baking.

—
Yield: 6 servings

PER SERVING: 218 calories (9% from fat, 50% from protein, 41% from carbohydrate); 27 g protein; 2 g total fat; 1 g saturated fat; 1 g monounsaturated fat; 1 g polyunsaturated fat; 22 g carbohydrate; 4 g fiber; 8 g sugar; 274 mg phosphorus; 70 mg calcium; 3 mg iron; 128 mg sodium; 766 mg potassium; 704 IU vitamin A; 7 mg ATE vitamin E; 26 mg vitamin C; 46 mg cholesterol; 239 g water

Turkey and Zucchini Meatloaf

The glaze gives this a nice sweet-tart taste. The turkey keeps it low in fat. The zucchini keeps it moist. What more could you ask?

1¼ pounds (570 g) ground turkey

1 cup (125 g) zucchini, grated

½ cup (60 g) low sodium bread crumbs

¼ cup (60 ml) egg substitute

1 tablespoon (0.4 g) dried parsley

½ teaspoon (1 g) black pepper

½ teaspoon (1.5 g) garlic powder

1 teaspoon (3 g) onion powder

¼ cup (80 g) peach preserves

2 teaspoons (10 g) Dijon mustard

Preheat oven to 350°F (180°C, or gas mark 4). Combine first 8 ingredients (through onion powder) in a large bowl and mix well. Shape mixture into a loaf on a baking sheet. Bake for 45 minutes. Stir preserves and mustard together. Spread on top of loaf. Return to the oven and bake for 20 minutes, or until the internal temperature is 165°F (74°C).

—

Yield: 8 servings

PER SERVING: 144 calories (12% from fat, 51% from protein, 37% from carbohydrate); 18 g protein; 2 g total fat; 1 g saturated fat; 0 g monounsaturated fat; 1 g polyunsaturated fat; 13 g carbohydrate; 1 g fiber; 6 g sugar; 162 mg phosphorus; 32 mg calcium; 2 mg iron; 126 mg sodium; 282 mg potassium; 100 IU vitamin A; 0 mg ATE vitamin E; 4 mg vitamin C; 52 mg cholesterol; 80 g water

Chicken Curry

I'm fond of curries. They make a particularly nice slow-cooker meal because they fill the house with such a great aroma for you to come home to. This one calls for a number of spices that are typical of curry powder. If you have a favorite curry powder on the shelf, you could substitute a couple of tablespoons of that for the other spices.

5 medium potatoes, diced

¾ cup (112 g) green bell peppers, coarsely chopped

¾ cup (120 g) onion, coarsely chopped

1 pound (455 g) boneless chicken breasts, cubed

2 cups (360 g) canned no-salt-added tomatoes

1 tablespoon (6 g) ground coriander

1½ tablespoons (10.5 g) paprika

1 tablespoon (5.5 g) ground ginger

¼ teaspoon (0.5 g) cayenne pepper

½ teaspoon (1.1 g) turmeric

¼ teaspoon (0.6 g) cinnamon

⅛ teaspoon (0.3 g) ground cloves

1 cup (235 ml) low sodium chicken broth

2 tablespoons (60 ml) cold water

¼ cup (32 g) cornstarch

Place potatoes, green bell peppers, and onion in slow cooker. Place chicken on top. Mix together tomatoes and the next 8 ingredients (through chicken broth). Pour over chicken. Cook on low 8 to 10 hours or on high 5 to 6 hours. Remove chicken and vegetables. Turn heat to high. Stir cornstarch into water. Add to cooker. Cook for 15 to 20 minutes, or until sauce is slightly thickened.

—
Yield: 5 servings

PER SERVING: 438 calories (5% from fat, 28% from protein, 67% from carbohydrate); 30 g protein; 2 g total fat; 1 g saturated fat; 0 g monounsaturated fat; 1 g polyunsaturated fat; 74 g carbohydrate; 8 g fiber; 8 g sugar; 448 mg phosphorus; 87 mg calcium; 5 mg iron; 126 mg sodium; 2235 mg potassium; 1394 IU vitamin A; 5 mg ATE vitamin E; 71 mg vitamin C; 53 mg cholesterol; 484 g water

Baked Chicken Nuggets

You can greatly reduce the amount of fat in chicken nuggets by baking them instead of frying them. The flavor is just as good, and they are a lot better for you.

½ cup (14 g) crushed corn flakes

2 tablespoons (15 g) nonfat dry milk

1 tablespoon (0.4 g) dried parsley

1 tablespoon (7 g) paprika

1 teaspoon (3 g) onion powder

¼ teaspoon (0.8 g) garlic powder

½ teaspoon (0.4 g) poultry seasoning

1 pound (455 g) boneless chicken breasts, cut in strips

¼ cup (60 ml) egg substitute

Preheat oven to 350°F (180°C, or gas mark 4). Mix together crushed corn flakes and next 6 ingredients (through poultry seasoning) in a resealable plastic bag. Dip chicken pieces in egg substitute, then place in bag. Shake to coat evenly. Place on baking sheet coated with nonstick vegetable oil spray. Bake for 20 minutes, or until chicken is done and coating is crispy.

—

Yield: 4 servings

PER SERVING: 167 calories (12% from fat, 73% from protein, 14% from carbohydrate); 29 g protein; 2 g total fat; 1 g saturated fat; 1 g monounsaturated fat; 1 g polyunsaturated fat; 6 g carbohydrate; 1 g fiber; 2 g sugar; 274 mg phosphorus; 61 mg calcium; 2 mg iron; 116 mg sodium; 442 mg potassium; 1088 IU vitamin A; 22 mg ATE vitamin E; 3 mg vitamin C; 66 mg cholesterol; 98 g water

Grilled Southwestern Chicken Breasts

The cilantro and lime give these chicken breasts a nice southwestern flavor.

4 boneless chicken breasts

¼ cup (60 ml) olive oil

2 tablespoons (30 g) Dijon mustard

1 tablespoon (15 ml) rice wine vinegar

1 teaspoon (2 g) black pepper

dash hot pepper sauce

¼ cup (60 ml) lime juice

2 tablespoons (8 g) cilantro

Pound the chicken breasts to ½-inch (1.3-cm) thickness and place all ingredients in a 1-gallon (3.8-L) resealable plastic bag or a bowl and cover. Marinate in the refrigerator for at least 30 minutes. Grill over medium heat for 20 minutes, or until done.

—
Yield: 4 servings

PER SERVING: 209 calories (64% from fat, 32% from protein, 4% from carbohydrate); 17 g protein; 15 g total fat; 2 g saturated fat; 10 g monounsaturated fat; 2 g polyunsaturated fat; 2 g carbohydrate; 0 g fiber; 0 g sugar; 151 mg phosphorus; 18 mg calcium; 1 mg iron; 133 mg sodium; 226 mg potassium; 117 IU vitamin A; 4 mg ATE vitamin E; 6 mg vitamin C; 41 mg cholesterol; 78 g water

TIP

Serve with rice and grilled corn.

Cajun Grilled Chicken

Nice Cajun flavor off the grill. Serve with rice and a steamed vegetable.

4 boneless chicken breasts

5 teaspoons (10 g) Cajun
blackening spice mix

—

Yield: 4 servings

Cut slashes into the chicken ½-inch (1.3-cm) deep to allow spices to penetrate the meat. Rub the spices into the chicken. Cook on a medium grill for about 25 minutes, or until done.

PER SERVING: 78 calories (11% from fat, 89% from protein, 0% from carbohydrate); 16 g protein; 1 g total fat; 0 g saturated fat; 0 g monounsaturated fat; 0 g polyunsaturated fat; 0 g carbohydrate; 0 g fiber; 0 g sugar; 139 mg phosphorus; 8 mg calcium; 1 mg iron; 46 mg sodium; 181 mg potassium; 15 IU vitamin A; 4 mg ATE vitamin E; 1 mg vitamin C; 41 mg cholesterol; 53 g water

Jerk Chicken Breasts

A simple recipe for jerk-flavored chicken. You could also cook this on the grill or a rotisserie.

½ cup (80 g) onion, finely chopped

6 boneless chicken breasts

1 teaspoon (2.5 g) paprika

2 teaspoons (6 g) garlic powder

3 tablespoons (19 g) jerk seasoning

—

Yield: 6 servings

Preheat oven to 350°F (180°C, or gas mark 4). Rub the onion into the chicken, inside and out. Combine the paprika, garlic powder, and jerk seasoning. Rub all over the chicken and allow the chicken to marinate for at least 2 hours. Roast in oven for 45 minutes to an hour, or until done.

PER SERVING: 88 calories (10% from fat, 80% from protein, 10% from carbohydrate); 17 g protein; 1 g total fat; 0 g saturated fat; 0 g monounsaturated fat; 0 g polyunsaturated fat; 2 g carbohydrate; 0 g fiber; 1 g sugar; 148 mg phosphorus; 12 mg calcium; 1 mg iron; 47 mg sodium; 220 mg potassium; 217 IU vitamin A; 4 mg ATE vitamin E; 2 mg vitamin C; 41 mg cholesterol; 65 g water

Smoked Turkey

If you have a smoker, this makes a sweet and juicy meal for a crowd, with a slightly southwestern flavor. Remember to discard the skin. It has most of the saturated fat, and it tends to get rubbery in the smoker anyway, so you're less tempted to cheat.

10-pound (4.5 kg) turkey

1 apple, quartered

1 onion, quartered

1 cup (100 g) celery, sliced

¼ cup (60 ml) honey

¼ cup (60 ml) lime juice

½ teaspoon (1.3 g) paprika

1 tablespoon (7 g) cumin

½ teaspoon (0.9 g) cayenne pepper

½ teaspoon (1.5 g) garlic powder

Place apple, onion, and celery inside turkey cavity. Combine remaining ingredients. Loosen the skin of the breast, legs, and thighs. Rub the honey spice mixture under the skin, spreading it as far as possible. Smoke for 8 to 10 hours, or until done.

—
Yield: 20 servings

PER SERVING: 271 calories (13% from fat, 79% from protein, 9% from carbohydrate); 51 g protein; 4 g total fat; 1 g saturated fat; 1 g monounsaturated fat; 1 g polyunsaturated fat; 6 g carbohydrate; 0 g fiber; 5 g sugar; 424 mg phosphorus; 35 mg calcium; 4 mg iron; 144 mg sodium; 634 mg potassium; 79 IU vitamin A; 0 mg ATE vitamin E; 2 mg vitamin C; 166 mg cholesterol; 191 g water

6

Beef Mains

Beef producers tell us that "it's what's for dinner," and I have to admit that in our household this was often true. We had beef three or four times a week. However, current dietary guidelines often recommend limiting yourself to no more than one or two meals a week of red meat. But that doesn't mean we need to give up the taste we love completely. The key is being selective about the cuts of beef that you buy. An ounce of chuck or prime rib contains over 6 grams of fat, but the same amount of round steak only has about 1 gram. Ground beef comes in a range of 5% fat to 20% fat, which is marked right on the package. The ground beef I buy, and what is specified in the following recipes, in 93% lean. You will need to be more careful how you cook your lean beef to get maximum flavor and tenderness out of it. The recipes in this chapter will show you how you can enjoy beef and still keep to your cholesterol–healthy diet.

Barbecued Beef

This is a quick sandwich meal that will cook while you are out. Small children and teenagers seem to like this too, so it's great for a party or family get-together.

1½ pounds (680 g) extra-lean ground beef (93% lean)

1 onion, chopped

1 cup (240 g) low sodium ketchup

1 green bell pepper, chopped

2 tablespoons (30 g) brown sugar

½ teaspoon (1.5 g) garlic powder

2 tablespoons (30 g) prepared mustard

3 tablespoons (45 ml) vinegar

1 tablespoon (15 ml) Worcestershire sauce

1 teaspoon (2.6 g) chili powder

In a skillet, brown beef and onion. Drain. Stir together remaining ingredients in slow cooker. Stir in meat and onion mixture. Cook on low for 6 to 8 hours or on high for 3 to 4 hours.

—
Yield: 8 servings

PER SERVING: 249 calories (32% from fat, 40% from protein, 28% from carbohydrate); 17 g protein; 6 g total fat; 2 g saturated fat; 2 g monounsaturated fat; 0 g polyunsaturated fat; 12 g carbohydrate; 0 g fiber; 10 g sugar; 135 mg phosphorus; 18 mg calcium; 2 mg iron; 85 mg sodium; 402 mg potassium; 377 IU vitamin A; 0 mg ATE vitamin E; 8 mg vitamin C; 59 mg cholesterol; 80 g water

Meatloaf

This meatloaf, with variations as our diet has changed, has been a family favorite for years. It's a simple loaf with only a few ingredients, which my kids seemed to appreciate. The sauce is the real star here, a sweet and sour barbecue-y marvel that is worlds away from plain tomato sauce or, heaven forbid, tomato soup. It gives the whole house a wonderful aroma while it cooks. I always make at least a double recipe. It makes great sandwiches. You can also use ground turkey and make a lower-fat version.

1½ pounds (680 g) extra-lean ground beef (93% lean)

1 cup (115 g) bread crumbs

1 onion, finely chopped

¼ cup (60 ml) egg substitute

¼ teaspoon (0.5 g) black pepper

8 ounces (225 g) no-salt-added tomato sauce, divided

½ cup (120 ml) water

2 teaspoons (10 ml) Worcestershire sauce

3 tablespoons (45 ml) vinegar

2 tablespoons (30 g) mustard

3 tablespoons (45 g) brown sugar

Preheat oven to 350°F (180°C, or gas mark 4). Mix together beef, bread crumbs, onion, egg substitute, pepper, and half the tomato sauce. Form into one large loaf or two small ones; mix remaining tomato sauce and remaining ingredients together; pour over loaves. Bake for 1 to 1½ hours.

—
Yield: 6 servings

PER SERVING: 393 calories (29% from fat, 37% from protein, 33% from carbohydrate); 26 g protein; 9 g total fat; 3 g saturated fat; 3 g monounsaturated fat; 1 g polyunsaturated fat; 23 g carbohydrate; 1 g fiber; 9 g sugar; 218 mg phosphorus; 62 mg calcium; 4 mg iron; 249 mg sodium; 585 mg potassium; 175 IU vitamin A; 0 mg ATE vitamin E; 8 mg vitamin C; 78 mg cholesterol; 142 g water

German Meatballs

These German-flavored meatballs would traditionally be served over spaetzle, but they are also good with noodles, rice, or mashed potatoes.

¼ cup (60 ml) egg substitute

¼ cup (60 ml) skim milk

¼ cup (29 g) bread crumbs

¼ teaspoon (0.2 g) poultry seasoning

1 pound (455 g) extra-lean
ground beef (93% lean)

2 cups (470 ml) low sodium
beef broth

½ cup (35 g) mushrooms, sliced

½ cup (80 g) onion, chopped

1 cup (230 g) fat-free sour cream

1 tablespoon (8 g) flour

1 teaspoon (2.1 g) caraway seed

Combine egg substitute and milk. Stir in bread crumbs and poultry seasoning. Add beef and mix well. Form into 24 meatballs, each about 1½ inches (3.8 cm). Brown meatballs in skillet. Drain. Add broth, mushrooms, and onion to the skillet. Cover and simmer for 30 minutes. Stir together sour cream, flour, and caraway seed. Add to skillet. Cook and stir until thickened.

—
Yield: 6 servings

PER SERVING: 281 calories (32% from fat, 47% from protein, 21% from carbohydrate); 19 g protein; 6 g total fat; 2 g saturated fat; 2 g monounsaturated fat; 1 g polyunsaturated fat; 8 g carbohydrate; 1 g fiber; 1 g sugar; 199 mg phosphorus; 87 mg calcium; 2 mg iron; 172 mg sodium; 417 mg potassium; 212 IU vitamin A; 47 mg ATE vitamin E; 2 mg vitamin C; 68 mg cholesterol; 194 g water

Stuffed Banana Peppers

Another recipe that uses some excess peppers. The original recipe I used to develop this one called for frying, but I decided to make them in the oven instead to reduce the amount of fat, since the meat and cheese already have a significant amount.

12 banana peppers, hot or sweet

1 pound (455 g) extra-lean ground beef (93% lean)

½ cup (80 g) onion, finely chopped

½ cup (55 g) Swiss cheese, shredded

¼ cup (60 ml) egg substitute

¼ teaspoon (0.5 g) black pepper

¼ cup (30 g) flour

Preheat oven to 350°F (180°C, or gas mark 4). Wash and clean peppers, then cut off the top and a small part of the bottom of peppers. In a large skillet, sauté ground beef and onions until meat is browned. Stir in cheese. Stuff mixture into peppers. Whisk egg substitute and black pepper in a bowl. Dip peppers in egg mixture. Roll in flour, dip in egg again, and roll in flour again. Place in 9 x 13-inch (23 x 33-cm) baking dish and coat surface with nonstick vegetable oil spray until flour is moistened. Bake for 20 minutes, or until cheese is melted and coating begins to brown.

—
Yield: 4 servings

PER SERVING: 372 calories (32% from fat, 47% from protein, 21% from carbohydrate); 30 g protein; 9 g total fat; 4 g saturated fat; 4 g monounsaturated fat; 1 g polyunsaturated fat; 14 g carbohydrate; 4 g fiber; 3 g sugar; 325 mg phosphorus; 195 mg calcium; 3 mg iron; 159 mg sodium; 685 mg potassium; 419 IU vitamin A; 7 mg ATE vitamin E; 83 mg vitamin C; 84 mg cholesterol; 204 g water

Chili Casserole

A Mexican meal in one pan. This is a fairly mild version, but you could increase the chili powder or add a chopped jalapeño to either the chili or the cornbread if you wanted to make it spicier.

1 pound (455 g) extra-lean ground beef (93% lean)

½ cup (80 g) onion, chopped

½ cup (75 g) red bell pepper, chopped

2 cups (450 g) no-salt-added kidney beans

2 cups (360 g) tomatoes, chopped and drained

1 cup (164 g) frozen corn

1 tablespoon (7.5 g) chili powder

1 teaspoon (2.5 g) cumin

½ teaspoon (1.5 g) garlic powder

½ cup (60 g) flour

½ cup (70 g) yellow cornmeal

2 tablespoons (26 g) sugar

1½ teaspoons (7 g) baking powder

1 cup (235 ml) skim milk

¼ cup (60 ml) egg substitute, or 1 egg

1 tablespoon (15 ml) olive oil

Preheat oven to 425°F (220°C, or gas mark 7). Brown beef with onions and red bell pepper until beef is no longer pink. Add beans, tomatoes, corn, chili powder, cumin, and garlic powder and simmer for 5 minutes. In a large bowl, stir together flour, cornmeal, sugar, and baking powder. In a medium bowl, combine milk, egg, and oil and pour into flour mixture, stirring until just moistened. Spread beef mixture in a greased 8 × 8-inch (20 × 20-cm) baking dish. Spread cornmeal mixture over top. Bake for 10 to 12 minutes, or until cornbread is done.

—
Yield: 4 servings

PER SERVING: 669 calories (20% from fat, 28% from protein, 52% from carbohydrate); 39 g protein; 13 g total fat; 4 g saturated fat; 6 g monounsaturated fat; 2 g polyunsaturated fat; 74 g carbohydrate; 13 g fiber; 10 g sugar; 506 mg phosphorus; 288 mg calcium; 8 mg iron; 357 mg sodium; 1247 mg potassium; 1838 IU vitamin A; 38 mg ATE vitamin E; 49 mg vitamin C; 80 mg cholesterol; 340 g water

Mexican Skillet Meal

This is one of those one-pan meals that you used to buy in a box. I have to say I think the flavor of this one is better than anything Hamburger Helper ever did.

1 pound (455 g) extra-lean ground beef (93% lean)

½ cup (80 g) onion, chopped

¼ cup (37 g) green bell peppers, chopped

¼ cup (37 g) red bell pepper, chopped

½ teaspoon (1.5 g) minced garlic

1½ cups (290 g) rice

3 cups (710 ml) water

2 teaspoons (4 g) low sodium beef bouillon

2 cups (360 g) canned no-salt-added tomatoes

1 tablespoon (7.5 g) chili powder

½ teaspoon (1.3 g) cumin

¼ teaspoon (0.3 g) dried oregano

12 ounces (340 g) frozen corn, thawed

Sauté beef, onion, green and red bell peppers, and garlic in a large skillet until beef is browned and vegetables are tender. Add rice and sauté 2 minutes longer. Stir in remaining ingredients. Bring to boil. Reduce heat, cover, and simmer for 20 minutes, or until rice is tender and liquid is absorbed.

—

Yield: 5 servings

PER SERVING: 357 calories (22% from fat, 31% from protein, 47% from carbohydrate); 22 g protein; 7 g total fat; 2 g saturated fat; 3 g monounsaturated fat; 1 g polyunsaturated fat; 33 g carbohydrate; 4 g fiber; 6 g sugar; 225 mg phosphorus; 64 mg calcium; 4 mg iron; 98 mg sodium; 653 mg potassium; 826 IU vitamin A; 0 mg ATE vitamin E; 29 mg vitamin C; 63 mg cholesterol; 404 g water

Enchilada Bake

An easy casserole dish with the taste of enchiladas.

1 pound (455 g) extra-lean ground beef (93% lean)

¼ cup (40 g) onion, chopped

1 cup (235 ml) egg substitute

8 ounces (225 g) no-salt-added tomato sauce

⅔ cup (160 ml) fat-free evaporated milk

2 tablespoons (5 g) taco seasoning

¼ cup (34 g) ripe olives, sliced

1 cup (28 g) corn chips

¾ cup (90 g) low fat cheddar cheese, shredded

Preheat oven to 350°F (180°C, or gas mark 4). In a skillet, cook beef and onion until meat is brown and onion is soft. Drain. Spread in the bottom of a 9-inch (23-cm) square baking dish that has been coated with nonstick vegetable oil spray. Beat together egg substitute, tomato sauce, milk, and taco seasoning. Pour over meat. Sprinkle with olives. Top with corn chips. Bake for 25 minutes, or until set in the center. Sprinkle cheese on top and return to oven just until cheese melts, about 3 minutes.

—

Yield: 6 servings

PER SERVING: 339 calories (38% from fat, 41% from protein, 22% from carbohydrate); 27 g protein; 11 g total fat; 3 g saturated fat; 4 g monounsaturated fat; 2 g polyunsaturated fat; 14 g carbohydrate; 1 g fiber; 6 g sugar; 322 mg phosphorus; 206 mg calcium; 3 mg iron; 455 mg sodium; 621 mg potassium; 586 IU vitamin A; 44 mg ATE vitamin E; 6 mg vitamin C; 57 mg cholesterol; 160 g water

Fall Stew

Apple cider gives this stew its unique flavor.

3 tablespoons (24 g) flour

¼ teaspoon (0.5 g) black pepper

¼ teaspoon (0.3 g) dried thyme

2 pounds (905 g) beef round steak,
cut in 1-inch (2.5-cm) cubes

3 tablespoons (45 ml) olive oil

2 cups (470 ml) apple cider

2 tablespoons (30 ml) cider vinegar

3 medium potatoes, peeled and quartered

1½ cups (195 g) carrot, sliced

1 cup (160 g) onion, quartered

½ cup (50 g) celery, sliced

Combine flour, pepper, and thyme. Dredge meat in flour mixture. Heat oil in Dutch oven. Brown half the meat at a time in the oil. Return all meat to the pan. Stir in cider and vinegar. Cook and stir until mixture boils. Reduce heat, cover and simmer 1¼ hours, or until the meat is tender. Stir in potatoes, carrot, onion, and celery. Cover and cook until vegetables are done, about 30 minutes more.

—
Yield: 8 servings

PER SERVING: 430 calories (24% from fat, 42% from protein, 34% from carbohydrate); 44 g protein; 11 g total fat; 3 g saturated fat; 6 g monounsaturated fat; 1 g polyunsaturated fat; 36 g carbohydrate; 3 g fiber; 10 g sugar; 361 mg phosphorus; 36 mg calcium; 5 mg iron; 89 mg sodium; 1193 mg potassium; 4077 IU vitamin A; 0 mg ATE vitamin E; 18 mg vitamin C; 102 mg cholesterol; 256 g water

Cabbage Beef Soup

This is one of those throw-together meals that turned out to be a keeper. It's quick and easy and has a lot of flavor.

½ pound (225 g) extra-lean ground beef (93% lean)

½ cup (80 g) onion, chopped

1 cup (70 g) cabbage, shredded

1 cup (180 g) canned no-salt-added tomatoes

2 cups (450 g) Mexican beans

1 cup (235 ml) water

Brown beef and onion in a large saucepan. Drain. Add cabbage and continue cooking until cabbage is soft, about 5 minutes. Add tomatoes, beans, and water. Bring to a boil and simmer 10 minutes to blend the flavors.

—
Yield: 5 servings

PER SERVING: 213 calories (16% from fat, 37% from protein, 47% from carbohydrate); 16 g protein; 3 g total fat; 1 g saturated fat; 1 g monounsaturated fat; 0 g polyunsaturated fat; 20 g carbohydrate; 8 g fiber; 2 g sugar; 179 mg phosphorus; 77 mg calcium; 4 mg iron; 44 mg sodium; 570 mg potassium; 76 IU vitamin A; 0 mg ATE vitamin E; 13 mg vitamin C; 31 mg cholesterol; 199 g water

TIP

For variety, replace the cabbage with packaged coleslaw or broccoli slaw mix.

Beef and Black Bean Stew

Not quite a chili, but with a definite southwestern flavor, this one is always a big hit at our house.

2 pounds (905 g) extra-lean ground beef (93% lean)

½ teaspoon (1.5 g) minced garlic

1 cup (160 g) onion, chopped

2 cups (360 g) canned no-salt-added tomatoes

1 cup (225 g) salsa

1 teaspoon (2.5 g) ground cumin

½ teaspoon (1 g) freshly ground black pepper

1 cup (170 g) frozen corn, thawed

2 cups (450 g) black beans, drained and rinsed

1 tablespoon (4 g) chopped fresh cilantro

In a large skillet, brown ground beef with garlic and onion. Drain and transfer to a slow cooker. Add tomatoes, salsa, cumin, pepper, corn, and black beans. Cook on low 6 to 8 hours or on high for 3 to 4 hours. Add cilantro during the last hour of cooking.

—

Yield: 8 servings

PER SERVING: 369 calories (28% from fat, 41% from protein, 32% from carbohydrate); 27 g protein; 8 g total fat; 3 g saturated fat; 3 g monounsaturated fat; 1 g polyunsaturated fat; 21 g carbohydrate; 6 g fiber; 4 g sugar; 268 mg phosphorus; 55 mg calcium; 4 mg iron; 282 mg sodium; 779 mg potassium; 238 IU vitamin A; 0 mg ATE vitamin E; 9 mg vitamin C; 78 mg cholesterol; 220 g water

TIP

To make a meal, top with grated cheese, guacamole, or sour cream, and serve with tortilla chips or cornbread.

Scottish Oxtail Soup

Oxtails may be difficult to find, although you might get some from an old-fashioned butcher or meat market. Here, in the metropolitan Washington, DC, area, I can occasionally get oxtails from the meat department at some of the big supermarkets.

1 bay leaf

2 tablespoons (4.8 g) fresh thyme

¼ cup (15 g) fresh parsley

½ cup (50 g) celery, chopped, plus one 4-inch (10-cm) piece celery stalk

2 scallions

4 cups (946 ml) low sodium beef broth

1 pound (455 g) oxtail, cut into pieces, fat removed

½ cup (80 g) onion, chopped

½ cup (65 g) carrot, chopped

4 ounces (115 g) no-salt-added tomato sauce

1 tablespoon (8 g) flour

3 tablespoons (45 ml) port wine

Make a spice bag by placing bay leaf, thyme, parsley (including stalks), one 4-inch (10-cm) piece celery stalk with leaves, and scallions in the center of a square of double thickness cheesecloth. Fold up the sides of the cheesecloth and tie off the top very tightly. Pour the beef broth into a saucepan and add the oxtail and onion, carrot, tomato sauce, and remaining celery, as well as the spice bag. Bring to a boil, and then transfer to a slow cooker and cook on high for 1½-2 hours (or longer if necessary) until the meat is tender. Strain the stock, cut all the meat from the bones and then return the stock and meat to the saucepan. Bring to a boil. Mix the flour and port together and add to the soup. Simmer for 5 minutes before serving.

—
Yield: 6 servings

PER SERVING: 148 calories (23% from fat, 56% from protein, 21% from carbohydrate); 19 g protein; 3 g total fat; 1 g saturated fat; 2 g monounsaturated fat; 0 g polyunsaturated fat; 7 g carbohydrate; 2 g fiber; 3 g sugar; 198 mg phosphorus; 63 mg calcium; 4 mg iron; 161 mg sodium; 566 mg potassium; 2187 IU vitamin A; 0 mg ATE vitamin E; 9 mg vitamin C; 29 mg cholesterol; 269 g water

7

Pork Mains

Like beef, pork used to be a staple of our diet. Growing up in a home with German heritage, pork was on our menu often, and that carried over to my adult life. And like beef, pork can contain a lot of saturated fat if you aren't careful about the cut. However, also like beef, there is good news out there. For the past few years, I've been able to find whole pork loins at stores for around USD $2.00 a pound. These can easily be cut into great tasting, lean chops, as well as into any size roast you want. And most of your favorite pork recipes can be adapted to use a cut from the loin instead of the fattier cuts you may have been used to. In this chapter, you'll find recipes not just for chops and roasts, but for everything from soups and stir-fries to your favorite barbecue recipes.

Hawaiian Kabobs

Serve these with rice for an island treat.

½ cup (120 ml) Reduced-Sodium Soy Sauce (see recipe page 15)

2 tablespoons (30 ml) olive oil

1 tablespoon (15 g) brown sugar

½ teaspoon (1.5 g) minced garlic

1 teaspoon (3 g) dry mustard

1 teaspoon (1.8 g) ground ginger

2 pounds (905 g) pork tenderloin, cut in 1-inch (2.5-cm) cubes

2 cups (300 g) green bell peppers, cut in 1-inch (2.5-cm) pieces

20 cherry tomatoes

6 ounces (170 g) pineapple chunks

In a large bowl combine soy sauce, oil, brown sugar, garlic, mustard, and ginger. Add pork cubes; cover and refrigerate overnight. Drain meat, reserving marinade. Thread meat, green bell pepper, tomatoes, and pineapple on skewers. Grill over medium-hot fire for 15 minutes, or until pork is done. Baste with marinade with cooking.

—
Yield: 6 servings

PER SERVING: 279 calories (11% from fat, 17% from protein, 72% from carbohydrate); 33 g protein; 10 g total fat; 2 g saturated fat; 6 g monounsaturated fat; 4 g polyunsaturated fat; 140 g carbohydrate; 2 g fiber; 8 g sugar; 370 mg phosphorus; 34 mg calcium; 2 mg iron; 217 mg sodium; 867 mg potassium; 566 IU vitamin A; 3 mg ATE vitamin E; 54 mg vitamin C; 98 mg cholesterol; 213 g water

Stir-Fried Pork and Cabbage

Not a traditional Asian stir-fry, but it still as an interesting flavor combination and is good served over rice.

1 pound (455 g) pork loin chops, sliced thinly

1 tablespoon (15 ml) olive oil

1 cup (150 g) apple, sliced thinly

3 tablespoons (45 ml) honey

4 cups (280 g) cabbage, shredded

Slice pork. Heat oil in wok or skillet, add pork and stir-fry until no longer pink, about 5 minutes. Add apples and honey, stir-fry 1 minute. Add cabbage and stir-fry for 30 to 45 seconds, or until heated through, but still crispy.

—
Yield: 4 servings

PER SERVING: 259 calories (28% from fat, 38% from protein, 33% from carbohydrate); 25 g protein; 8 g total fat; 2 g saturated fat; 5 g monounsaturated fat; 1 g polyunsaturated fat; 22 g carbohydrate; 3 g fiber; 19 g sugar; 274 mg phosphorus; 53 mg calcium; 2 mg iron; 75 mg sodium; 604 mg potassium; 106 IU vitamin A; 2 mg ATE vitamin E; 35 mg vitamin C; 71 mg cholesterol; 192 g water

Apple Cranberry Stuffed Pork Roast

When I said I was going to make this, my wife wondered about going to the trouble of butterflying the roast, but the results were worth what turned out to be not a lot of effort. This is the kind of meal you could serve to anyone without worrying that it seems like a special "diet" food.

⅔ cup (160 ml) apple cider

¼ cup (60 ml) cider vinegar

½ cup (115 g) light brown sugar, packed

1 tablespoon (0.9 g) dried shallots

1 cup (86 g) dried apples

½ cup (75 g) dried cranberries

1 teaspoon (1.8 g) ground ginger

½ teaspoon (1.9 g) mustard seed

½ teaspoon (0.8 g) ground allspice

⅛ teaspoon (0.3 g) cayenne pepper

2 pounds (905 g) boneless
pork loin roast

—
Yield: 8 servings

PER SERVING: 269 calories (26% from fat, 38% from protein, 37% from carbohydrate); 25 g protein; 8 g total fat; 3 g saturated fat; 3 g monounsaturated fat; 1 g polyunsaturated fat; 24 g carbohydrate; 1 g fiber; 22 g sugar; 245 mg phosphorus; 24 mg calcium; 1 mg iron; 58 mg sodium; 581 mg potassium; 41 IU vitamin A; 2 mg ATE vitamin E; 1 mg vitamin C; 62 mg cholesterol; 121 g water

Combine all ingredients except pork in medium saucepan and bring to a simmer over medium-high heat. Cover; reduce heat to low, and cook until apples are very soft, about 20 minutes. Strain through a fine-mesh sieve, using a rubber spatula to press against the apple mixture in the sieve to extract as much liquid as possible; reserve the liquid. Return liquid to saucepan and simmer over medium-high heat until reduced to ½ cup (120 ml), about 5 minutes. Remove from heat, set aside, and reserve for use as a glaze.

Preheat oven to 350°F (180°C, or gas mark 4) or prepare your grill for indirect heat. Lay the roast down, fat side up. Insert a knife into the roast ½ inch (1.3 cm) horizontally from the bottom of the roast, along the long side of the roast. Make a long cut along the bottom of the roast, stopping ½ inch (1.3 cm) before the edge of the roast. You might find it easier to handle by starting at a corner of the roast. Open up the roast and continue to cut through the thicker half of the roast, again keeping ½ inch (1.3 cm) from the bottom. Repeat until the roast is an even ½-inch (1.3-cm) thickness all over when laid out. Spread out the filling on the roast, leaving a ½-inch (1.3-cm) border from the edges. Starting with the short side of the roast, roll it up very tightly. Secure with kitchen twine at 1-inch (2.5-cm) intervals. If baking, place the roast on a rack in a roasting pan and cook on the middle rack of the oven. If you are grilling using indirect heat, preheat the grill and wipe the grates with olive oil. Place roast, fat side up, on the side of the grill that has no coals underneath. Cover the grill with the lid. Cook for 45 to 60 minutes (if you are grilling, turn roast halfway through the cooking). Brush the roast with half of the glaze and cook for 5 minutes longer. Remove the roast from the oven or grill. Place it on a cutting board. Cover with foil to rest and keep warm for 15 minutes before slicing. Slice into ½-inch (1.3-cm) pieces, removing the cooking twine as you cut the roast. Serve with remaining glaze.

Glazed Pork Roast

You can also grill this using indirect heat. Place a pan of water under the roast and mound the charcoal around it. Close the grill. This makes excellent sandwiches, too.

¼ cup (60 ml) honey

1 tablespoon (9 g) dry mustard

¼ cup (60 ml) white wine vinegar

1 teaspoon (2.6 g) chili powder

2 pounds (905 g) pork tenderloin

Preheat oven to 350°F (180°C, or gas mark 4). Mix together the first 4 ingredients. Trim excess fat from pork roast. Brush with honey glaze. Roast for 1 to 1½ hours, or until done, brushing with additional glaze occasionally.

—

Yield: 8 servings

PER SERVING: 173 calories (22% from fat, 57% from protein, 21% from carbohydrate); 24 g protein; 4 g total fat; 1 g saturated fat; 2 g monounsaturated fat; 0 g polyunsaturated fat; 9 g carbohydrate; 0 g fiber; 9 g sugar; 258 mg phosphorus; 9 mg calcium; 2 mg iron; 61 mg sodium; 436 mg potassium; 101 IU vitamin A; 2 mg ATE vitamin E; 1 mg vitamin C; 74 mg cholesterol; 94 g water

Stuffed Pork Roast

This pork loin is filled with a traditional cornbread stuffing. If you put a drip pan under the roast during the indirect cooking phase and add some water to it, you will end up with the makings of a delicious gravy. Remember not to let the drip pan dry out.

2 tablespoons (30 ml) olive oil

½ cup (160 g) onion, chopped

1 teaspoon (3 g) minced garlic

1 tablespoon (2 g) dried sage, chopped

4 cups (600 g) Lower-Fat Cornbread, cubed (see recipe page 126)

¼ cup (60 ml) egg substitute

1 cup (235 ml) low sodium chicken broth

2 pounds (905 g) pork loin roast

In a skillet, heat oil over medium-high heat. Add onions and garlic and cook until tender. Add sage and cook for about 30 seconds. Remove from heat and add cornbread, onion mixture, and egg substitute. Stir, adding the chicken broth slowly until it becomes spreadable (it should look like stuffing). Butterfly the pork loin. Spread stuffing over the pork loin and roll up. Secure with kitchen twine at 1-inch (2.5-cm) intervals. Preheat grill and prepare for indirect grilling. Place pork loin on grill over direct heat. Turn every two minutes until the surface of the pork loin is seared. Move to indirect portion of grill and continue cooking for about 30 minutes or until the meat reaches an internal temperature of 155°F (68°C). Remove from grill and let rest for 5 minutes. Slice and serve.

—

Yield: 8 servings

PER SERVING: 371 calories (31% from fat, 38% from protein, 31% from carbohydrate); 28 g protein; 10 g total fat; 3 g saturated fat; 6 g monounsaturated fat; 2 g polyunsaturated fat; 24 g carbohydrate; 3 g fiber; 4 g sugar; 303 mg phosphorus; 53 mg calcium; 2 mg iron; 222 mg sodium; 552 mg potassium; 391 IU vitamin A; 75 mg ATE vitamin E; 3 mg vitamin C; 72 mg cholesterol; 193 g water

Pork Loin Roast

This pork roast has a Latin flavor. The sauce is good over rice or noodles.

3 pounds (1.4 kg) pork loin roast

1 tablespoon (7.5 g) chili powder

½ cup (120 ml) lime juice

1 teaspoon (2.5 g) cumin

1 teaspoon (1 g) dried oregano

½ teaspoon (1 g) black pepper

½ teaspoon (1.5 g) minced garlic

6 ounces (170 g) orange juice concentrate, thawed, divided

¼ cup (60 ml) dry white wine

½ cup (115 g) fat-free sour cream

Place pork roast in a shallow glass dish. Mix chili powder, lime juice, cumin, oregano, pepper, garlic, and ¼ cup (60 ml) of orange juice concentrate and brush mixture onto the pork roast. Cover and refrigerate at least 8 hours. Preheat oven to 325°F (170°C, or gas mark 3). Place pork on a rack in a shallow roasting pan. Roast uncovered for 1½ to 2 hours, or until thermometer registers 170°F (77°C). Remove pork and rack from the pan. Strain the drippings from the pan and set aside. Add enough water to remaining orange juice concentrate to measure ¾ cup (180 ml); stir juice and wine into the drippings, then stir in the sour cream. Serve with the pork roast.

—
Yield: 9 servings

PER SERVING: 255 calories (26% from fat, 57% from protein, 17% from carbohydrate); 33 g protein; 7 g total fat; 2 g saturated fat; 3 g monounsaturated fat; 1 g polyunsaturated fat; 10 g carbohydrate; 1 g fiber; 7 g sugar; 361 mg phosphorus; 49 mg calcium; 2 mg iron; 93 mg sodium; 748 mg potassium; 397 IU vitamin A; 16 mg ATE vitamin E; 32 mg vitamin C; 100 mg cholesterol; 151 g water

Pork Loin Roast with Asian Vegetables

Serve this Asian-style pork roast with rice for a complete meal.

1 teaspoon (1.8 g) ground ginger

2 tablespoons (30 ml) olive oil

2 pounds (905 g) pork loin roast

1¼ cups (295 ml) water, divided

1 cup (160 g) onion, coarsely chopped

¼ cup (60 ml) Reduced-Sodium
Soy Sauce (see recipe page 15)

¼ cup (60 ml) red wine vinegar

2 tablespoons (30 g) brown sugar

½ teaspoon (1.5 g) garlic powder

¼ teaspoon (0.5 g) black pepper

4 cups (250 g) snow pea pods

2 cups (360 g) canned no-salt-added
tomatoes, undrained

8 ounces (225 g) water chestnuts

1 cup mushrooms (70 g), sliced

2 tablespoons (16 g) cornstarch

In a large Dutch oven, sauté ginger in oil for 30 seconds. Add pork roast and brown meat on all sides. Add 1 cup (235 ml) water, onion, soy sauce, vinegar, brown sugar, garlic powder, and pepper. Cover and simmer for 1½ hours, or until tender. Add pea pods, tomatoes and liquid, water chestnuts, and mushrooms. Cover and simmer for 3 to 5 minutes, or until crisp-tender. Remove vegetables and meat. Skim any fat from pan juices. Blend the remaining ¼ cup (60 ml) water with the cornstarch and stir into the pot. Cook and stir until bubbly. Serve sauce with vegetables and meat.

—
Yield: 8 servings

PER SERVING: 273 calories (16% from fat, 23% from protein, 60% from carbohydrate); 27 g protein; 8 g total fat; 2 g saturated fat; 5 g monounsaturated fat; 2 g polyunsaturated fat; 70 g carbohydrate; 3 g fiber; 10 g sugar; 325 mg phosphorus; 72 mg calcium; 3 mg iron; 128 mg sodium; 893 mg potassium; 615 IU vitamin A; 2 mg ATE vitamin E; 39 mg vitamin C; 71 mg cholesterol; 285 g water

Italian Pork Roast

This can be part of a great Italian meal, but it also makes the best Italian pork sub sandwiches that you will ever have.

½ teaspoon (1 g) ground allspice

1 teaspoon (2 g) fennel seed, crushed

1 teaspoon (1.2 g) dried rosemary

1 teaspoon (2 g) black pepper

2½ pound (1.1 kg) pork loin roast

Preheat oven to 325°F (170°C, or gas mark 3). Combine allspice, fennel, rosemary, and pepper and mix well. Rub this mixture thoroughly into all sides of the roast. Marinate in the refrigerator overnight. Bake for 30 to 40 minutes per pound, until internal temperature is 170°F (77°C).

—
Yield: 8 servings

PER SERVING: 42 calories (31% from fat, 66% from protein, 4% from carbohydrate); 7 g protein; 1 g total fat; 0 g saturated fat; 1 g monounsaturated fat; 0 g polyunsaturated fat; 0 g carbohydrate; 0 g fiber; 0 g sugar; 71 mg phosphorus; 9 mg calcium; 0 mg iron; 17 mg sodium; 126 mg potassium; 6 IU vitamin A; 1 mg ATE vitamin E; 0 mg vitamin C; 20 mg cholesterol; 23 g water

Winter Pork Stew

One of those meals that just takes too long to fix when you get home from work, transformed into an easy slow-cooker creation.

4 sweet potatoes, peeled and sliced

2 pounds (905 g) pork loin roast

½ cup (115 g) brown sugar

¼ teaspoon (0.5 g) cayenne pepper

¼ teaspoon (0.5 g) black pepper

¼ teaspoon (0.8 g) garlic powder

½ teaspoon (1.5 g) onion powder

Place sweet potatoes in the bottom of a slow cooker. Place pork on top. Combine remaining ingredients and sprinkle over pork and potatoes. Cover and cook on low 8 to 10 hours. Remove pork and slice. Serve juices over pork and potatoes.

—
Yield: 8 servings

PER SERVING: 256 calories (18% from fat, 40% from protein, 43% from carbohydrate); 25 g protein; 5 g total fat; 2 g saturated fat; 2 g monounsaturated fat; 1 g polyunsaturated fat; 27 g carbohydrate; 2 g fiber; 18 g sugar; 276 mg phosphorus; 48 mg calcium; 2 mg iron; 84 mg sodium; 645 mg potassium; 11915 IU vitamin A; 2 mg ATE vitamin E; 11 mg vitamin C; 71 mg cholesterol; 144 g water

Pork Chops with Red Cabbage

Make your own sweet-and-sour red cabbage while cooking flavorful pork chops.

4 cups (280 g) red cabbage, shredded

½ cup (80 g) onion, chopped

1 apple, peeled and chopped

½ cup (115 g) brown sugar

½ cup (120 ml) cider vinegar

4 pork loin chops

Place cabbage, onion, and apple in a slow cooker. Combine sugar and vinegar, pour over vegetables and stir to mix. Place pork chops on top of mixture. Cook on low for 7 to 8 hours.

—

Yield: 4 servings

PER SERVING: 290 calories (14% from fat, 32% from protein, 55% from carbohydrate); 23 g protein; 4 g total fat; 2 g saturated fat; 2 g monounsaturated fat; 1 g polyunsaturated fat; 40 g carbohydrate; 3 g fiber; 34 g sugar; 265 mg phosphorus; 85 mg calcium; 2 mg iron; 89 mg sodium; 765 mg potassium; 1013 IU vitamin A; 2 mg ATE vitamin E; 54 mg vitamin C; 64 mg cholesterol; 229 g water

Barbecued Pork

This recipe for pulled pork is made in the oven, but it could also be cooked in a smoker or using indirect heat on a grill.

3 pounds (1.4 kg) pork loin roast

1 teaspoon (1.2 g) red pepper flakes

1 teaspoon (2 g) black pepper

1 cup (235 ml) apple cider

1 cup (235 ml) apple cider vinegar

1 cup (160 g) onion, sliced

½ teaspoon (1.5 g) minced garlic

Preheat oven to 300°F (160°C, or gas mark 2). Coat a large baking pan with nonstick vegetable oil spray. Rub the pork with the red pepper flakes and pepper and place in the prepared baking pan. Pour the cider and vinegar over and around the pork. Scatter the onions and garlic over and around the pork. Cover with aluminum foil. Roast for 3 hours. Uncover and continue to roast for 1 hour, or until an instant-read thermometer inserted into the thickest part of the pork registers 180°F (82°C). Remove the pork from the oven and transfer to a plate. Let stand for 1 hour. Using two forks, shred the pork by steadying the meat with one fork and pulling it away with the other, discarding any fat.

—

Yield: 12 servings

PER SERVING: 165 calories (28% from fat, 62% from protein, 10% from carbohydrate); 24 g protein; 5 g total fat; 2 g saturated fat; 2 g monounsaturated fat; 1 g polyunsaturated fat; 4 g carbohydrate; 0 g fiber; 3 g sugar; 255 mg phosphorus; 22 mg calcium; 1 mg iron; 60 mg sodium; 484 mg potassium; 70 IU vitamin A; 2 mg ATE vitamin E; 2 mg vitamin C; 71 mg cholesterol; 132 g water

Pork Chops with Scalloped Potatoes

Real comfort food—pork chops and potatoes baked together in a flavorful sauce.

3 tablespoons (45 ml) canola oil, divided

3 tablespoons (24 g) flour

¼ teaspoon (0.5 g) black pepper

2 cups (470 ml) low sodium chicken broth

6 pork loin chops, ¾-inch (1.9-cm) thick

6 medium potatoes, thinly sliced

1 cup (160 g) onion, sliced

—
Yield: 6 servings

Preheat oven to 350°F (180°C, or gas mark 4). In a saucepan, heat 2 tablespoons (30 ml) oil, stir in flour and pepper. Add chicken broth; cook and stir constantly until mixture boils. Cook for 1 minute; remove from heat and set aside. In a skillet, brown pork chops in remaining 1 tablespoon (15 ml) oil. In a greased 9 × 13-inch (23 × 33-cm) baking dish, layer potatoes and onion. Pour the broth mixture over. Place pork chops on top. Cover and bake for 1 hour; uncover and bake 30 minutes longer, or until potatoes are tender.

PER SERVING: 624 calories (24% from fat, 34% from protein, 42% from carbohydrate); 52 g protein; 17 g total fat; 4 g saturated fat; 8 g monounsaturated fat; 3 g polyunsaturated fat; 65 g carbohydrate; 6 g fiber; 6 g sugar; 692 mg phosphorus; 63 mg calcium; 4 mg iron; 164 mg sodium; 2489 mg potassium; 49 IU vitamin A; 4 mg ATE vitamin E; 42 mg vitamin C; 127 mg cholesterol; 479 g water

Pork and Apple Curry

Curry flavor creates a new kind of pork dish.

2 tablespoons (30 ml) olive oil

4 pork loin chops

½ cup (80 g) onion, thinly sliced

¼ teaspoon (0.8 g) minced garlic

1 apple, peeled and sliced

½ cup (75 g) red bell pepper, cut in strips

½ cup (120 ml) low sodium chicken broth

1 teaspoon (2 g) cornstarch

1 teaspoon (2 g) curry powder

½ teaspoon (1.3 g) ground cumin

½ teaspoon (1.2 g) cinnamon

¼ teaspoon (0.5 g) freshly ground black pepper

In a heavy frying pan, heat oil over medium-high heat. Cook pork chops until browned on both sides and almost cooked through; remove from pan and set aside. Over medium heat, cook the onion, garlic, apple, and red bell pepper strips for 2 minutes or until softened. Blend chicken broth with cornstarch; add to pan along with curry powder, cumin, and cinnamon; cook for 1 or 2 minutes, or until slightly reduced and thickened. Return pork chops to frying pan. Cook for 1 or 2 minutes or until heated through. Serve pork chops with sauce and sprinkle with pepper.

—
Yield: 4 servings

PER SERVING: 228 calories (45% from fat, 39% from protein, 15% from carbohydrate); 23 g protein; 11 g total fat; 3 g saturated fat; 7 g monounsaturated fat; 1 g polyunsaturated fat; 9 g carbohydrate; 2 g fiber; 5 g sugar; 247 mg phosphorus; 31 mg calcium; 2 mg iron; 63 mg sodium; 513 mg potassium; 612 IU vitamin A; 2 mg ATE vitamin E; 28 mg vitamin C; 64 mg cholesterol; 166 g water

TIP

Serve with quick-cooking couscous flavored with chopped scallions and raisins.

Caribbean Grilled Pork

Grilled pork, seasoned with a spicy sauce. The pork tenderloin is low in fat, but still very tender. Be careful not to overcook.

2 pounds (905 g) pork tenderloin

½ cup (120 ml) bottled jerk sauce

—

Yield: 4 servings

Make shallow cuts in the roast and rub in the sauce. Marinate overnight. Grill at lowest possible setting for 15 to 20 minutes, or until done. Adding apple or other aromatic wood to the fire will add to the flavor.

PER SERVING: 307 calories (24% from fat, 65% from protein, 11% from carbohydrate); 48 g protein; 8 g total fat; 3 g saturated fat; 4 g monounsaturated fat; 1 g polyunsaturated fat; 8 g carbohydrate; 0 g fiber; 6 g sugar; 516 mg phosphorus; 14 mg calcium; 3 mg iron; 144 mg sodium; 878 mg potassium; 68 IU vitamin A; 5 mg ATE vitamin E; 2 mg vitamin C; 147 mg cholesterol; 184 g water

8

Soups, Stews, and Chilis

I love soups and stews, especially during cooler weather. And the moist, slow cooking in a Dutch oven or slow cooker can turn even the leanest cuts of meat into tender morsels. They tend to make very healthy meals, low in fat, full of other good nutrition, and often needing only a slice of bread to make a complete meal. In this chapter, you'll find all the traditional favorite soups, as well as a selection of recipes with flavors from around the globe and a few that probably have never been seen anywhere else.

Amish Chicken Soup

When I was growing up along the Maryland/Pennsylvania border, Amish chicken corn soup was always one of the highlights at volunteer fire company carnivals and suppers. This soup has a similar flavor.

4 cups (946 ml) low sodium chicken broth

2 cups (220 g) chicken, cooked and chopped

½ cup (50 g) celery, chopped

½ cup (65 g) carrot, sliced

½ cup (80 g) onion, chopped

1 tablespoon (0.4 g) dried parsley

¼ teaspoon (0.8 g) garlic powder

2 cups (470 ml) water

12 ounces (340 g) egg noodles

Place all ingredients in a large kettle and simmer until noodles are tender (see package directions for approximate time).

—
Yield: 8 servings

PER SERVING: 148 calories (22% from fat, 37% from protein, 41% from carbohydrate); 14 g protein; 4 g total fat; 1 g saturated fat; 1 g monounsaturated fat; 1 g polyunsaturated fat; 15 g carbohydrate; 3 g fiber; 1 g sugar; 144 mg phosphorus; 20 mg calcium; 1 mg iron; 49 mg sodium; 262 mg potassium; 1456 IU vitamin A; 6 mg ATE vitamin E; 2 mg vitamin C; 31 mg cholesterol; 248 g water

Ham and Bean Soup

Bean soup is one of those classic comfort foods. Add a big slice of dark bread and everything is right with your world.

1 pound (455 g) dried navy beans

8 cups (1.9 L) water

½ pound (225 g) ham, cubed

2 medium potatoes, peeled and cubed

½ cup (50 g) celery, sliced

½ cup (65 g) carrots, sliced

½ cup (80 g) onion, chopped

¼ teaspoon (0.5 g) black pepper

Soak beans in water overnight. Do not drain. Bring beans to a boil in the soaking liquid. Add ham, reduce heat, cover, and simmer for 1 hour or until beans are nearly done. Add remaining ingredients, cover, and simmer for 30 minutes more, or until vegetables are done.

—

Yield: 10 servings

PER SERVING: 148 calories (13% from fat, 26% from protein, 61% from carbohydrate); 10 g protein; 2 g total fat; 1 g saturated fat; 1 g monounsaturated fat; 0 g polyunsaturated fat; 23 g carbohydrate; 4 g fiber; 2 g sugar; 162 mg phosphorus; 42 mg calcium; 2 mg iron; 464 mg sodium; 594 mg potassium; 1104 IU vitamin A; 0 mg ATE vitamin E; 8 mg vitamin C; 9 mg cholesterol; 313 g water

Caribbean Turkey Soup

This makes a flavorful soup that is also a good way to use up leftover holiday turkey.

1½ pounds (680 g) turkey breast, cut into bite-sized pieces

1 teaspoon (2.5 g) paprika

1 cup (160 g) onion, coarsely chopped

½ cup (75 g) green bell pepper, coarsely chopped

½ teaspoon (1.5 g) finely chopped garlic

1 cup (100 g) celery, coarsely chopped

½ cup (35 g) mushrooms, sliced

2 cups (360 g) canned no-salt-added tomatoes

1 cup (235 ml) low sodium chicken broth

1 cup (134 g) frozen peas, thawed

¼ teaspoon (0.5 g) black pepper

¼ teaspoon (0.3 g) dried thyme

2 medium potatoes, peeled and chopped

1 tablespoon (0.4 g) dried parsley

¼ teaspoon (0.3 g) dried oregano

In a large skillet or saucepan, combine turkey and paprika. Cook over medium heat, about 5 minutes. Remove turkey and set aside. Place onions, green bell pepper, garlic, celery, and mushrooms in skillet. Cook, stirring, about 4 minutes. Add remaining ingredients; mix well. Add turkey; cook, covered, over low heat about 40 minutes.

—
Yield: 6 servings

PER SERVING: 277 calories (8% from fat, 47% from protein, 45% from carbohydrate); 33 g protein; 3 g total fat; 1 g saturated fat; 0 g monounsaturated fat; 1 g polyunsaturated fat; 31 g carbohydrate; 6 g fiber; 6 g sugar; 379 mg phosphorus; 77 mg calcium; 4 mg iron; 203 mg sodium; 1274 mg potassium; 1044 IU vitamin A; 0 mg ATE vitamin E; 34 mg vitamin C; 68 mg cholesterol; 376 g water

Winter Vegetable Soup

A good meal for a winter's evening. With no potatoes or pasta, it's also low in carbohydrates for an entire meal. Using a lean cut of meat like round steak also makes it low in fat.

1 pound (455 g) beef round steak

2 cups (470 ml) low sodium beef broth

2 cups (360 g) canned no-salt-added tomatoes

1 cup (150 g) turnips, diced

6 ounces (170 g) frozen green beans, thawed

6 ounces (170 g) frozen broccoli, thawed

6 ounces (170 g) frozen cauliflower, thawed

½ cup (65 g) carrot, sliced

½ cup (80 g) onion, diced

½ cup (50 g) celery, diced

Combine all ingredients in a slow cooker and cook on low for 8 to 10 hours or high 4 to 5 hours. Remove meat and cut into bite-sized pieces or shred. Return to slow cooker and stir until warmed through.

—
Yield: 4 servings

PER SERVING: 317 calories (19% from fat, 59% from protein, 23% from carbohydrate); 47 g protein; 7 g total fat; 2 g saturated fat; 2 g monounsaturated fat; 1 g polyunsaturated fat; 18 g carbohydrate; 7 g fiber; 8 g sugar; 377 mg phosphorus; 119 mg calcium; 6 mg iron; 188 mg sodium; 1135 mg potassium; 3451 IU vitamin A; 0 mg ATE vitamin E; 82 mg vitamin C; 102 mg cholesterol; 493 g water

Beef Goulash

This is the kind of stew that has been popular in the United States since colonial days. And with good reason—you couldn't ask for a better cold-weather meal.

5 tablespoons (40 g) flour, divided

¼ teaspoon (0.5 g) black pepper

2 pounds (905 g) beef round steak, cut in 1-inch (2.5-cm) cubes

2 tablespoons (30 ml) olive oil

1½ cups (240 g) onion, sliced

1 cup (235 ml) apple juice

1⅓ cups (320 ml) water, divided

4 cups (560 g) rutabagas, cut in 1-inch (2.5-cm) cubes

3 cups (390 g) carrot, sliced

½ teaspoon (0.1 g) dried parsley

½ teaspoon (0.3 g) dried marjoram

½ teaspoon (0.5 g) dried thyme

6 potatoes, peeled, cooked, and mashed

Combine 2 tablespoons (16 g) of the flour with the pepper in a resealable plastic bag. Add meat a little at a time and shake to coat. Brown the meat in the oil in a Dutch oven, half at a time. Return all meat to Dutch oven, add onions, juice, and 1 cup (235 ml) of the water. Cover and simmer about 1¼ hours, or until meat is tender. Add rutabagas, carrot, parsley, marjoram, and thyme. Cover and simmer about 30 minutes more, until vegetables are done. Blend the remaining ⅓ cup (80 ml) water and the remaining 3 tablespoons (24 g) of the flour and stir into stew. Cook and stir until thickened and bubbly. Spoon mashed potatoes around the edge of the stew to serve.

—
Yield: 8 servings

PER SERVING: 538 calories (16% from fat, 36% from protein, 48% from carbohydrate); 48 g protein; 10 g total fat; 3 g saturated fat; 5 g monounsaturated fat; 1 g polyunsaturated fat; 64 g carbohydrate; 9 g fiber; 14 g sugar; 499 mg phosphorus; 94 mg calcium; 7 mg iron; 120 mg sodium; 2117 mg potassium; 8103 IU vitamin A; 0 mg ATE vitamin E; 47 mg vitamin C; 102 mg cholesterol; 489 g water

Italian Kitchen Sink Soup

Okay, so the name's kind of strange. But it sure seems like it has everything in it. In truth, it's a heartier version of the Italian Wedding Soup that's become popular in recent years. This one is truly a meal in a bowl. And it's low in fat and sodium, but high in fiber and vitamins.

4 cups (946 ml) water

2 cups (320 g) onion, chopped

2 red potatoes, diced

1 cup (250 g) dried great northern beans

½ cup (65 g) carrot, sliced

½ cup (35 g) mushrooms, sliced

½ cup (100 g) uncooked pearl barley

½ pound (225 g) round steak, cubed

2 cups (360 g) canned no-salt-added tomatoes

2 cups (470 ml) low sodium beef broth

1 tablespoon (2.1 g) Italian seasoning

½ teaspoon (1.5 g) minced garlic

1 cup (113 g) zucchini, sliced

1 cup (20 g) fresh spinach, torn into bite-sized pieces

½ cup (75 g) small pasta

1 tablespoon (3.3 g) dried rosemary

½ teaspoon (1 g) black pepper

Combine first 12 ingredients (through garlic) in a large electric slow cooker. Cover with lid, and cook on high for 6 hours or low for 10 to 12 hours. Add remaining ingredients, cover and cook on high-heat setting for an additional 30 minutes, or until beans are tender.

—
Yield: 8 servings

PER SERVING: 209 calories (9% from fat, 30% from protein, 61% from carbohydrate); 16 g protein; 2 g total fat; 1 g saturated fat; 1 g monounsaturated fat; 0 g polyunsaturated fat; 33 g carbohydrate; 8 g fiber; 4 g sugar; 203 mg phosphorus; 112 mg calcium; 4 mg iron; 256 mg sodium; 689 mg potassium; 4349 IU vitamin A; 0 mg ATE vitamin E; 15 mg vitamin C; 18 mg cholesterol; 366 g water

Savory Beef Stew

Here is the kind of meal you need as the weather starts to turn cooler (seems like I say that about a lot of recipes!). It has a wonderful aroma and flavor, thanks to a couple of unusual ingredients. And it can cook while you're away, so it's ready when you arrive home.

2 tablespoons (16 g) flour

1 pound (455 g) beef round steak, cubed

2 tablespoons (30 ml) olive oil

4 medium potatoes, cubed

1 cup (130 g) carrot, sliced

½ cup (80 g) onion, coarsely chopped

1 cup (235 ml) low sodium beef broth

2 cups (360 g) canned no-salt-added tomatoes

½ cup (120 ml) water

2 tablespoons (30 g) brown sugar

1 tablespoon (15 ml) Worcestershire sauce

1 tablespoon (15 ml) vinegar

1½ teaspoons (1.5 g) instant coffee

1 teaspoon (2.5 g) cumin

½ teaspoon (0.9 g) ground ginger

¼ teaspoon (0.5 g) ground allspice

Place flour in a plastic bag. Add beef and shake to coat. Heat oil in a large skillet over medium heat. Brown beef on all sides. Place potatoes, carrots, and onion in a slow cooker. Top with beef. Combine remaining ingredients and pour over meat and vegetables. Cover and cook on low for 8 to 10 hours or on high 4 to 5 hours.

—
Yield: 6 servings

PER SERVING: 424 calories (19% from fat, 32% from protein, 49% from carbohydrate); 34 g protein; 9 g total fat; 2 g saturated fat; 5 g monounsaturated fat; 1 g polyunsaturated fat; 53 g carbohydrate; 6 g fiber; 10 g sugar; 361 mg phosphorus; 74 mg calcium; 6 mg iron; 126 mg sodium; 1682 mg potassium; 3705 IU vitamin A; 0 mg ATE vitamin E; 35 mg vitamin C; 68 mg cholesterol; 413 g water

Pork Stew

It's nice to have dinner finished when you get home once in a while. You can serve this over rice or noodles or just have it with a big slice of freshly baked bread (the delay bake option on the bread machine works **so** well with the slow cooker).

1 pound (455 g) pork loin

¾ cup (120 g) onion, sliced

2 cups (360 g) canned no-salt-added tomatoes

½ cup (75 g) green bell pepper, coarsely chopped

2 cups (470 ml) low sodium chicken broth

1 cup (70 g) mushrooms, quartered

1 tablespoon (0.4 g) dried parsley

1 teaspoon (1 g) dried thyme

¼ cup (15 g) fresh cilantro, chopped

¼ cup (30 g) flour

Cube pork. Layer all ingredients except the flour in a slow cooker, reserving half the chicken broth. Cook on low for 6 to 8 hours. Stir the flour into the remaining chicken broth. Add to slow cooker. Turn to high and cook an additional 30 minutes, or until slightly thickened.

—
Yield: 4 servings

PER SERVING: 242 calories (35% from fat, 35% from protein, 30% from carbohydrate); 22 g protein; 10 g total fat; 4 g saturated fat; 4 g monounsaturated fat; 1 g polyunsaturated fat; 18 g carbohydrate; 3 g fiber; 70 mg calcium; 3 mg iron; 91 mg sodium; 801 mg potassium; 1073 IU vitamin A; 54 mg vitamin C; 52 mg cholesterol

Mock Crab Soup

This soup is typical of Maryland crab soup in flavor. The only big difference is the lack of crab meat, which is high in both sodium and cholesterol. In its place we have fish. I happened to have some flounder fillets available, but any white fish would do. This is also one of our spicier recipes. You can reduce the amount of pepper if you prefer a milder version.

1 pound (455 g) flounder

2 cups (470 ml) low sodium chicken broth

2 cups (360 g) canned no-salt-added tomatoes, diced

½ cup (82 g) frozen corn, thawed

½ cup (67 g) frozen peas, thawed

1½ teaspoons (3 g) seafood seasoning

½ teaspoon (1 g) black pepper

½ teaspoon (0.9 g) cayenne pepper

Shred the fish (processing in a food processor with a little of the broth does this easily). Place all ingredients in a large saucepan and simmer for 10 minutes, or until fish and vegetables are cooked.

—
Yield: 4 servings

PER SERVING: 178 calories (12% from fat, 58% from protein, 30% from carbohydrate); 26 g protein; 2 g total fat; 1 g saturated fat; 1 g monounsaturated fat; 1 g polyunsaturated fat; 14 g carbohydrate; 3 g fiber; 5 g sugar; 298 mg phosphorus; 70 mg calcium; 2 mg iron; 242 mg sodium; 810 mg potassium; 742 IU vitamin A; 11 mg ATE vitamin E; 16 mg vitamin C; 54 mg cholesterol; 350 g water

Fish Chowder

This makes a great chowder, thick and rich. You can substitute other fish, or a combination of different types of fish, for the cod.

2 tablespoons (30 ml) olive oil

2 cups (320 g) chopped onion

½ cup (35 g) mushrooms, sliced

½ cup (50 g) celery, chopped

5 cups (1.2 L) low sodium chicken broth, divided

4 medium potatoes, diced

2 pounds (905 g) cod, diced into ½-inch (1.3-cm) cubes

⅛ teaspoon (0.3 g) seafood seasoning

¼ teaspoon (0.5 g) black pepper

½ cup (60 g) flour

3 cups (710 ml) fat-free evaporated milk

In a large stockpot, heat oil over medium heat. Sauté onions, mushrooms, and celery until tender. Add 4 cups (946 ml) chicken broth and potatoes; simmer for 10 minutes. Add fish, and simmer another 10 minutes. Season to taste with seafood seasoning and pepper. Mix together remaining broth and flour until smooth; stir into soup. Cook until slightly thickened. Remove from heat and stir in evaporated milk.

—

Yield: 8 servings

PER SERVING: 397 calories (13% from fat, 35% from protein, 52% from carbohydrate); 35 g protein; 6 g total fat; 1 g saturated fat; 3 g monounsaturated fat; 1 g polyunsaturated fat; 52 g carbohydrate; 4 g fiber; 15 g sugar; 600 mg phosphorus; 334 mg calcium; 3 mg iron; 236 mg sodium; 1854 mg potassium; 468 IU vitamin A; 127 mg ATE vitamin E; 21 mg vitamin C; 53 mg cholesterol; 508 g water

Caribbean Fish Stew

This is a fairly spicy stew if you use the habanero pepper. I use a jalapeño instead, which still gives you some heat, but in moderation.

½ cup (65 g) carrot, sliced

1 cup (160 g) onion, sliced

2 tablespoons (28 g) grated fresh ginger

½ teaspoon (1.5 g) minced garlic

½ teaspoon (1 g) ground cloves

½ teaspoon (1 g) ground allspice

½ teaspoon (1 g) cardamom

½ teaspoon (1.1 g) turmeric

2 teaspoons (4 g) ground coriander

4 cups (360 g) canned no-salt-added tomatoes

12 ounces (355 ml) beer

1 habanero or jalapeño pepper

2 medium potatoes, diced

1 pound tilapia (455 g) fillets, cut into 2-inch (5-cm) pieces

1 tablespoon (4 g) cilantro, chopped

½ cup (120 ml) lime juice

In a Dutch oven, sauté the carrot and onion until slightly soft, then add the ginger and garlic. When the vegetables are soft, add the cloves, allspice, cardamom, turmeric, and coriander and sauté about 1 minute longer. Add the tomatoes and beer and bring to a boil. Add the habanero pepper. Reduce the heat and let simmer for 20 minutes, then add the potatoes. When the potatoes are tender, add the fish. Cook another 5 minutes. Then add the cilantro and lime juice. Stir and serve.

—
Yield: 4 servings

PER SERVING: 395 calories (9% from fat, 32% from protein, 59% from carbohydrate); 31 g protein; 4 g total fat; 1 g saturated fat; 1 g monounsaturated fat; 1 g polyunsaturated fat; 56 g carbohydrate; 8 g fiber; 11 g sugar; 454 mg phosphorus; 181 mg calcium; 6 mg iron; 131 mg sodium; 2078 mg potassium; 3282 IU vitamin A; 53 mg ATE vitamin E; 59 mg vitamin C; 36 mg cholesterol; 589 g water

Basic Chili

I never seem to make chili the same way twice, so I keep coming up with new recipes. One thing that's become fairly constant, though, is sautéing the spices, which seems to give it a deeper flavor.

1 pound (455 g) dried kidney beans

2 pounds (905 g) beef round steak

1 tablespoon (15 ml) olive oil

½ cup (80 g) onion, coarsely chopped

½ teaspoon (1.5 g) minced garlic

½ cup (75 g) green bell pepper, coarsely chopped

4 ounces (115 g) canned jalapeño peppers

2 tablespoons (15 g) chili powder

1 tablespoon (7 g) cumin

1 teaspoon (1 g) dried oregano

1 tablespoon (4 g) cilantro

2 cups (360 g) canned no-salt-added tomatoes

2 cups (360 g) canned no-salt-added crushed tomatoes

Soak kidney beans overnight. Drain and add fresh water. Simmer for 1½ hours, or until almost tender. Coarsely grind beef or chop into small cubes no bigger than ½ inch (1.3 cm). Heat oil in a skillet and sauté beef, onion, garlic, green bell pepper, and jalapeños until beef is browned on all sides. Add chili powder, cumin, oregano, and cilantro and sauté an additional 5 minutes. Transfer to slow cooker. Stir in tomatoes. Drain beans and add to slow cooker. Stir to mix, cover, and cook on low 4 to 5 hours.

—
Yield: 8 servings

PER SERVING: 353 calories (22% from fat, 54% from protein, 24% from carbohydrate); 48 g protein; 8 g total fat; 2 g saturated fat; 4 g monounsaturated fat; 1 g polyunsaturated fat; 21 g carbohydrate; 6 g fiber; 4 g sugar; 379 mg phosphorus; 77 mg calcium; 8 mg iron; 223 mg sodium; 948 mg potassium; 884 IU vitamin A; 0 mg ATE vitamin E; 28 mg vitamin C; 102 mg cholesterol; 249 g water

Black Bean and Squash Chili

Winter squash adds color and a seasonal twist to this vegetarian chili.

1 medium butternut squash

1 tablespoon (15 ml) olive oil

1 cup (160 g) onion, chopped

½ teaspoon (1.5 g) minced garlic

¾ cup (112 g) green bell pepper, chopped

4 cups (900 g) canned black beans, drained and rinsed

4 cups (720 g) canned no-salt-added tomatoes

4 ounces (115 g) canned chili peppers

1 teaspoon (2.5 g) ground cumin

½ teaspoon (0.5 g) dried oregano

Cut squash in half and scoop out and discard seeds. Place squash in a microwave-safe container with ¼-inch (63 mm) of water. Cover and microwave until tender, allowing 2 to 3 minutes per squash half. Remove squash and let cool, then peel and cut into chunks. In a large pot, heat oil over medium heat. Add onion and cook, stirring often, for 5 minutes or until soft. Add remaining ingredients except squash and mix well. Bring to a boil. Reduce heat and simmer gently for 15 minutes. Stir in squash and heat through.

—
Yield: 10 servings

PER SERVING: 199 calories (11% from fat, 17% from protein, 72% from carbohydrate); 9 g protein; 3 g total fat; 0 g saturated fat; 1 g monounsaturated fat; 1 g polyunsaturated fat; 39 g carbohydrate; 12 g fiber; 10 g sugar; 167 mg phosphorus; 92 mg calcium; 4 mg iron; 28 mg sodium; 951 mg potassium; 9267 IU vitamin A; 0 mg ATE vitamin E; 66 mg vitamin C; 0 mg cholesterol; 247 g water

9

Salads and Salad Dressings

Salads can be one of those good-news, bad-news kind of things when you are watching your diet. The salad itself is often very healthy, but the dressing may not be. You'll need to be careful about what kind of fat is in that bottle you pick up off the grocer's shelf. Many contain 2 to 3 grams of saturated fat and as much as 15 grams of total fat per serving. I've provided some tasty alternatives here with less than half that. There also are recipes for some meal-sized salads, side salads that aren't just the same old thing, and reduced-fat versions of favorites like potato salad.

Mexican Bean Salad

A simple and tasty South-of-the-border bean salad. Cook dry beans according to package directions or drain canned beans.

2 cups (450 g) cooked kidney beans

2 cups (450 g) cooked garbanzo beans

1 cup (180 g) tomatoes, chopped

¾ cup (105 g) cucumber, peeled and chopped

2 tablespoons (20 g) onion, diced

½ cup (115 g) avocado, mashed

½ cup (115 g) plain fat-free yogurt

¼ teaspoon (0.8 g) minced garlic

½ teaspoon (1.3 g) cumin

4 cups (80 g) lettuce, shredded

In a large bowl, toss together the kidney beans, garbanzo beans, tomatoes, cucumber, and onion. In a small bowl, mix the avocado, yogurt, garlic, and cumin. Stir the avocado mixture into the bean mixture and chill. Serve on top of shredded lettuce.

—
Yield: 8 servings

PER SERVING: 172 calories (17% from fat, 19% from protein, 64% from carbohydrate); 9 g protein; 3 g total fat; 0 g saturated fat; 2 g monounsaturated fat; 1 g polyunsaturated fat; 29 g carbohydrate; 7 g fiber; 2 g sugar; 164 mg phosphorus; 75 mg calcium; 3 mg iron; 303 mg sodium; 506 mg potassium; 346 IU vitamin A; 0 mg ATE vitamin E; 11 mg vitamin C; 0 mg cholesterol; 159 g water

Chicken Main-Dish Salad

A meal-on-a-plate. This makes a good hot weather dinner when you don't really feel like doing much cooking

FOR DRESSING:

6 tablespoons (90 ml) olive oil

¼ teaspoon (0.8 g) minced garlic

1 tablespoon (15 ml) lemon juice

2 tablespoons (30 ml) red wine vinegar

½ teaspoon (2.5 ml) Worcestershire sauce

FOR SALAD:

1 pound (455 g) boneless chicken breasts

12 ounces (340 g) romaine lettuce

1 cup (30 g) croutons

¼ cup (25 g) Parmesan cheese, grated

¼ teaspoon (0.5 g) freshly ground black pepper

Combine dressing ingredients in a jar with a tight-fitting lid and shake well. Place half of dressing in a resealable plastic bag with chicken breasts and marinate several hours. Remove chicken and discard dressing. Grill chicken until done and slice into strips. Place lettuce on plates and top with chicken. Add croutons, sprinkle with cheese and pepper. Serve with remaining dressing.

—
Yield: 4 servings

PER SERVING: 290 calories (44% from fat, 43% from protein, 13% from carbohydrate); 31 g protein; 14 g total fat; 3 g saturated fat; 8 g monounsaturated fat; 2 g polyunsaturated fat; 9 g carbohydrate; 2 g fiber; 1 g sugar; 304 mg phosphorus; 117 mg calcium; 2 mg iron; 235 mg sodium; 531 mg potassium; 4992 IU vitamin A; 14 mg ATE vitamin E; 25 mg vitamin C; 71 mg cholesterol; 178 g water

Asian-Flavored Chicken Salad

A great use for leftover chicken, whether roasted, grilled, or smoked.

6 cups (120 g) iceberg lettuce, torn into bite-sized pieces

¼ cup (25 g) scallions, sliced

½ cup (30 g) cilantro, chopped

½ cup (30 g) fresh parsley, chopped

½ cup (50 g) celery, sliced

¼ cup (60 ml) rice vinegar

1 tablespoon (15 ml) sesame oil

¼ cup (60 ml) Reduced-Sodium Soy Sauce (see recipe page 15)

1 tablespoon (8 g) sesame seeds

2 cups (220 g) cooked chicken breast, chopped

½ cup (100 g) mandarin oranges

¼ cup (31 g) slivered almonds

Chop lettuce, scallions, cilantro, parsley, and celery and toss together. For dressing, combine vinegar, sesame oil, soy sauce, and sesame seeds. Marinate the chopped chicken in the dressing for a few hours or overnight. Just before serving, add oranges, almonds, and chicken with dressing to salad. Toss well.

—

Yield: 4 servings

PER SERVING: 247 calories (15% from fat, 16% from protein, 68% from carbohydrate); 25 g protein; 11 g total fat; 2 g saturated fat; 5 g monounsaturated fat; 5 g polyunsaturated fat; 108 g carbohydrate; 3 g fiber; 8 g sugar; 253 mg phosphorus; 89 mg calcium; 2 mg iron; 188 mg sodium; 608 mg potassium; 1935 IU vitamin A; 4 mg ATE vitamin E; 27 mg vitamin C; 60 mg cholesterol; 241 g water

Tofu Salad

Fresh Asian-style vegetables and tofu along with an Asian dressing give this main-dish salad a different kind of flavor.

FOR SALAD:

½ pound (225 g) lettuce, shredded

4 ounces (115 g) snow peas

½ cup (65 g) carrot, shredded

1 cup (70 g) cabbage, shredded

½ cup (35 g) mushrooms, sliced

½ cup (75 g) red bell pepper, sliced

4 ounces (115 g) mung bean sprouts

½ cup (90 g) tomato, sliced

12 ounces (340 g) tofu, drained and cubed

FOR DRESSING:

1 tablespoon (15 ml) rice vinegar

2 tablespoons (30 ml) sesame oil

3 tablespoons (45 ml) Reduced-Sodium Soy Sauce (see recipe page 15)

2 cloves garlic, crushed

1 tablespoon (8 g) sesame seeds

½ teaspoon (0.9 g) ground ginger

TO MAKE THE SALAD: Toss salad ingredients.

TO MAKE THE DRESSING: Combine dressing ingredients and spoon dressing over salad.

—
Yield: 6 servings

PER SERVING: 111 calories (19% from fat, 7% from protein, 75% from carbohydrate); 5 g protein; 6 g total fat; 1 g saturated fat; 2 g monounsaturated fat; 4 g polyunsaturated fat; 57 g carbohydrate; 3 g fiber; 5 g sugar; 92 mg phosphorus; 55 mg calcium; 1 mg iron; 72 mg sodium; 365 mg potassium; 2728 IU vitamin A; 0 mg ATE vitamin E; 38 mg vitamin C; 0 mg cholesterol; 185 g water

Coleslaw

This makes a fairly sour slaw, which is just fine with me, especially if you are planning to put it on barbecue sandwiches. You could add more sugar or a little honey if you like it sweeter.

2 cups (140 g) cabbage, shredded

⅓ cup (40 g) carrot, shredded

¼ cup (56 g) low fat mayonnaise

¼ cup (60 g) fat-free sour cream

2 tablespoons (30 ml) vinegar

2 tablespoons (26 g) sugar

¼ teaspoon (0.5 g) celery seed

¼ teaspoon (0.8 g) onion powder

Stir dressing ingredients together. Pour over cabbage and stir to mix.

—
Yield: 6 servings

PER SERVING: 75 calories (46% from fat, 5% from protein, 49% from carbohydrate); 1 g protein; 3 g total fat; 1 g saturated fat; 0 g monounsaturated fat; 0 g polyunsaturated fat; 8 g carbohydrate; 1 g fiber; 6 g sugar; 27 mg phosphorus; 28 mg calcium; 0 mg iron; 95 mg sodium; 97 mg potassium; 1281 IU vitamin A; 10 mg ATE vitamin E; 11 mg vitamin C; 7 mg cholesterol; 52 g water

Reduced-Fat Potato Salad

Time for a little picnic stuff. Feel free to vary the vegetables to whatever suits you best.

6 medium potatoes

½ cup (115 g) low fat mayonnaise

¼ cup (60 g) fat-free sour cream

2 teaspoons (6 g) dry mustard

1 teaspoon (3 g) onion powder

2 tablespoons (30 ml) honey

½ teaspoon (1 g) black pepper

1 tablespoon (0.4 g) dried parsley

½ teaspoon (1 g) celery seed

¼ teaspoon (0.3 g) dried dill

¼ cup (37 g) green bell pepper, chopped

¼ cup (25 g) celery, sliced

½ cup (65 g) carrot, sliced

Boil potatoes until done. Rinse in cold water and allow to cool. Mix together mayonnaise, sour cream, mustard, onion powder, honey, black pepper, parsley, celery seed, and dill. Pour over potatoes and stir to coat. Fold in green bell pepper, celery, and carrot.

TIP

Unless you have very small potatoes to boil whole, cut them into smaller pieces before cooking.

—
Yield: 6 servings

PER SERVING: 371 calories (18% from fat, 8% from protein, 74% from carbohydrate); 8 g protein; 7 g total fat; 1 g saturated fat; 0 g monounsaturated fat; 0 g polyunsaturated fat; 69 g carbohydrate; 7 g fiber; 11 g sugar; 256 mg phosphorus; 63 mg calcium; 3 mg iron; 198 mg sodium; 1778 mg potassium; 1993 IU vitamin A; 10 mg ATE vitamin E; 39 mg vitamin C; 11 mg cholesterol; 339 g water

Tomato Pasta Salad

A cool and pleasing side dish with a simple dressing.

2 cups (300 g) dried pasta

1 cup (230 g) fat-free sour cream

¼ cup (60 ml) skim milk

1 tablespoon (4 g) fresh dill

1 tablespoon (15 ml) vinegar

½ teaspoon (1 g) black pepper

2 cups (270 g) cucumber, chopped

2 cups (360 g) tomatoes, chopped

Cook pasta in boiling salted water until al dente. Drain and rinse in cold water. Transfer cooked pasta to a large serving bowl. In a separate bowl, mix together sour cream, milk, dill, vinegar, and pepper. Set dressing aside. Mix cucumbers and tomatoes into the pasta. Pour dressing over pasta mixture and toss thoroughly to combine. Cover, and refrigerate at least 1 hour and preferably overnight. Stir just before serving.

—
Yield: 8 servings

PER SERVING: 91 calories (9% from fat, 19% from protein, 72% from carbohydrate); 3 g protein; 1 g total fat; 0 g saturated fat; 0 g monounsaturated fat; 0 g polyunsaturated fat; 11 g carbohydrate; 1 g fiber; 1 g sugar; 76 mg phosphorus; 57 mg calcium; 1 mg iron; 23 mg sodium; 211 mg potassium; 409 IU vitamin A; 35 mg ATE vitamin E; 11 mg vitamin C; 19 mg cholesterol; 92 g water

Garbanzo and Pasta Salad

Garbanzo beans can be purchased dried or canned. If using dried beans, cook according to package directions. For canned beans, be sure to drain and rinse them before using.

4 ounces (115 g) pasta

2 cups (480 g) cooked garbanzo beans

½ cup (75 g) red bell pepper, chopped

⅓ cup (33 g) celery, sliced

⅓ cup (43 g) carrot, sliced

¼ cup (25 g) scallions, chopped

3 tablespoons (45 ml) balsamic vinegar

2 tablespoons (28 g) low fat mayonnaise

2 teaspoons (10 g) mustard

½ teaspoon (1 g) black pepper

¼ teaspoon (0.2 g) dried Italian seasoning

4 cups (80 g) leaf lettuce, torn into bite-sized pieces

Cook pasta according to directions, omitting salt. Drain and rinse well under cold water until pasta is cool; drain well. Combine pasta, garbanzo beans, red bell pepper, celery, carrot, and scallions in medium bowl. Whisk together vinegar, mayonnaise, mustard, black pepper, and Italian seasoning in small bowl until blended. Pour over salad; toss to coat evenly. Cover and refrigerate up to 8 hours. Arrange lettuce on individual plates. Spoon salad over lettuce.

—
Yield: 8 servings

PER SERVING: 150 calories (16% from fat, 15% from protein, 69% from carbohydrate); 6 g protein; 3 g total fat; 0 g saturated fat; 0 g monounsaturated fat; 1 g polyunsaturated fat; 26 g carbohydrate; 4 g fiber; 1 g sugar; 103 mg phosphorus; 39 mg calcium; 1 mg iron; 226 mg sodium; 239 mg potassium; 2589 IU vitamin A; 2 mg ATE vitamin E; 18 mg vitamin C; 13 mg cholesterol; 87 g water

TIP

This recipe can also be used as a vegetarian main dish, yielding 4 servings.

10

Low Fat Baking

Baked goods tend to be high in fat. Sometimes it's the good kind of fat like canola oil, but more often it's the undesirable kind like solid shortening. However, there are ways to improve that situation. Many of the muffins and other baked goods here are fat-free. One key trick is to replace the oil in recipes with applesauce or strained baby fruit. This gives you baked goods with the same texture as their higher-fat cousins. Depending on the other ingredients, you may not be able to taste the difference at all. In some cases, like the apple and peach muffins, the fruit actually complements and adds to the flavor. There also are some reduced-fat versions here of baked goods that usually contain significant amounts of solid shortening, such as biscuits and cornbread.

Apple Butter Muffins

Sweet enough to eat without adding any toppings.

2 cups (250 g) flour

1 tablespoon (13.8 g) baking powder

2 tablespoons (25 g) sugar

5 tablespoons (70 g) unsalted margarine

¼ cup (60 ml) egg substitute

½ cup (120 ml) skim milk

6 tablespoons (90 ml) apple butter, divided

2 tablespoons (30 g) brown sugar

1 tablespoon (8 g) flour

¼ teaspoon (0.6 g) cinnamon

Preheat oven to 400°F (200°C, or gas mark 6). Combine flour, baking powder, and sugar in a mixing bowl. Cut in margarine until mixture resembles coarse crumbs. Combine egg substitute, milk, and 2 tablespoons (30 ml) of the apple butter. Stir until just moistened. Spoon into 12 paper-lined or greased muffin cups. Top each with 1 teaspoon (5 ml) of the apple butter. Combine brown sugar, flour, and cinnamon and sprinkle over the top. Bake for 20 to 25 minutes.

—
Yield: 12 servings

PER SERVING: 161 calories (29% from fat, 8% from protein, 63% from carbohydrate); 3 g protein; 5 g total fat; 1 g saturated fat; 2 g monounsaturated fat; 2 g polyunsaturated fat; 25 g carbohydrate; 1 g fiber; 8 g sugar; 68 mg phosphorus; 93 mg calcium; 1 mg iron; 140 mg sodium; 77 mg potassium; 251 IU vitamin A; 51 mg ATE vitamin E; 0 mg vitamin C; 0 mg cholesterol; 22 g water

Banana Strawberry Wheat Muffins

These are a seasonal sort of thing, good with fresh strawberries.

1 cup (125 g) flour

½ cup (60 g) whole wheat flour

¼ cup (50 g) sugar

¼ cup (28 g) wheat germ

2½ teaspoons (11.5 g) baking powder

½ teaspoon (2.3 g) baking soda

¼ cup (60 ml) egg substitute

¾ cup (180 ml) skim milk

⅓ cup (80 ml) canola oil

½ cup (110 g) banana, mashed

½ cup (85 g) strawberries, chopped

Preheat oven to 350°F (180°C, or gas mark 4). Stir together the first 6 ingredients (through baking soda). Mix together the rest of the ingredients and stir into the dry ingredients, stirring until just moistened. Spoon into greased or paper-lined muffin tins. Bake for 20 to 25 minutes, or until done.

—
Yield: 12 servings

PER SERVING: 157 calories (39% from fat, 10% from protein, 52% from carbohydrate); 4 g protein; 7 g total fat; 1 g saturated fat; 4 g monounsaturated fat; 2 g polyunsaturated fat; 21 g carbohydrate; 2 g fiber; 6 g sugar; 104 mg phosphorus; 87 mg calcium; 1 mg iron; 173 mg sodium; 142 mg potassium; 60 IU vitamin A; 9 mg ATE vitamin E; 5 mg vitamin C; 0 mg cholesterol; 33 g water

Tropical Muffins

For those mornings when you are trying to escape the last cold, wet days of winter, these muffins make it a little easier to picture Hawaii.

1¾ cups (215 g) flour

¼ cup (60 g) brown sugar

2½ teaspoons (11.5 g) baking powder

¼ cup (60 ml) egg substitute

¾ cup (180 ml) skim milk

⅓ cup (80 ml) applesauce

6 ounces (170 g) crushed pineapple with syrup, drained

¼ cup (18 g) flaked dried coconut

Preheat oven to 400°F (200°C, or gas mark 6). In a medium bowl, stir together flour, brown sugar, and baking powder. Combine egg substitute, milk, and applesauce and add to dry ingredients. Stir until just mixed. Stir in pineapple and coconut. Spoon into muffin cups lined with paper or coated with nonstick vegetable oil spray. Bake for 20 to 25 minutes.

—
Yield: 12 servings

PER SERVING: 112 calories (7% from fat, 11% from protein, 81% from carbohydrate); 3 g protein; 1 g total fat; 1 g saturated fat; 0 g monounsaturated fat; 0 g polyunsaturated fat; 23 g carbohydrate; 1 g fiber; 7 g sugar; 68 mg phosphorus; 90 mg calcium; 1 mg iron; 123 mg sodium; 106 mg potassium; 57 IU vitamin A; 9 mg ATE vitamin E; 1 mg vitamin C; 0 mg cholesterol; 39 g water

Streusel Muffins

These muffins are relatively low fat as well as low sodium, and they taste like old-fashioned coffee cake.

FOR STREUSEL:

½ cup (115 g) brown sugar

2 tablespoons (16 g) flour

2 teaspoons (4.6 g) cinnamon

FOR MUFFINS:

1½ cups (188 g) flour

½ cup (100 g) sugar

2 teaspoons (9.6 g) baking powder

¼ cup (56 g) unsalted margarine

½ cup (120 ml) skim milk

¼ cup (60 ml) egg substitute

TO MAKE THE STREUSEL: Stir together brown sugar, flour, and cinnamon. Set aside.

TO MAKE THE MUFFINS: Preheat oven to 375°F (190°C, or gas mark 5). Stir together flour, sugar, and baking powder. Cut in margarine until mixture resembles coarse crumbs. Combine milk and egg substitute. Add to dry ingredients and stir until just mixed. Divide half the batter evenly among 12 greased or paper-lined muffin cups. Sprinkle with half the streusel topping. Top with remaining batter and then remaining streusel topping. Bake for 20 to 25 minutes.

—
Yield: 12 servings

PER SERVING: 172 calories (21% from fat, 7% from protein, 72% from carbohydrate); 3 g protein; 4 g total fat; 1 g saturated fat; 2 g monounsaturated fat; 1 g polyunsaturated fat; 31 g carbohydrate; 1 g fiber; 17 g sugar; 58 mg phosphorus; 81 mg calcium; 1 mg iron; 142 mg sodium; 92 mg potassium; 241 IU vitamin A; 52 mg ATE vitamin E; 0 mg vitamin C; 0 mg cholesterol; 16 g water

Banana Bread

Another good recipe for using up bananas. This makes a great breakfast or snack.

1¾ cups (215 g) flour

1¼ teaspoons (5.8 g) baking powder

1 teaspoon (4.6 g) baking soda

⅔ cup (133 g) sugar

¼ cup (56 g) unsalted margarine

½ cup (120 ml) egg substitute

¼ cup (60 ml) skim milk

1 cup (225 g) mashed banana

¼ cup (30 g) chopped pecans

Preheat oven to 350°F (180°C, or gas mark 4). Stir together flour, baking powder, and baking soda. In a mixing bowl, cream sugar and margarine with an electric mixer until light and fluffy. Add egg substitute and milk, beating until smooth. Add dry ingredients and banana alternately, beating until smooth after each addition. Stir in pecans. Pour batter into lightly greased 9 × 4 × 2-inch (23 × 10 × 5-cm) loaf pan. Bake for 60 to 65 minutes, or until a knife inserted near the center comes out clean. Cool 10 minutes before removing from pan.

—

Yield: 12 servings

PER SERVING: 187 calories (28% from fat, 8% from protein, 64% from carbohydrate); 4 g protein; 6 g total fat; 1 g saturated fat; 3 g monounsaturated fat; 1 g polyunsaturated fat; 30 g carbohydrate; 1 g fiber; 14 g sugar; 61 mg phosphorus; 49 mg calcium; 1 mg iron; 219 mg sodium; 145 mg potassium; 261 IU vitamin A; 49 mg ATE vitamin E; 2 mg vitamin C; 0 mg cholesterol; 30 g water

Pumpkin Bread

If you have some leftover pumpkin when you make pumpkin pie, you can make it into pumpkin bread. This makes a great breakfast without even needing to put any toppings on it.

3 cups (600 g) sugar

1 cup (235 ml) applesauce

1 cup (235 ml) egg substitute

16 ounces canned or cooked fresh pumpkin

3½ cups (438 g) flour

4 teaspoons (18.4 g) baking soda

1 teaspoon (4.6 g) baking powder

2 teaspoons (4.6 g) cinnamon

1 teaspoon (1.8 g) ground ginger

⅔ cup (160 ml) water

Preheat oven to 350°F (180°C, or gas mark 4). Cream sugar and applesauce. Add egg substitute and pumpkin; mix well. Sift together flour, baking soda, baking powder, cinnamon, and ginger. Add to pumpkin mixture alternately with water. Mix well after each addition. Divide batter evenly between two well-greased and floured glass 9 × 5-inch (23 × 12.5-cm) loaf pans. Bake for 1½ hours, or until knife inserted near center comes out clean. Let stand for 10 minutes. Remove from pans to cool.

—
Yield: 24 servings

PER SERVING: 184 calories (3% from fat, 7% from protein, 90% from carbohydrate); 3 g protein; 1 g total fat; 0 g saturated fat; 0 g monounsaturated fat; 0 g polyunsaturated fat; 42 g carbohydrate; 1 g fiber; 27 g sugar; 44 mg phosphorus; 28 mg calcium; 1 mg iron; 250 mg sodium; 103 mg potassium; 2983 IU vitamin A; 0 mg ATE vitamin E; 1 mg vitamin C; 0 mg cholesterol; 43 g water

Banana Sticky Buns

Am I the only one that seems to always have bananas at that use-or-throw-away stage? I hate throwing things away, so I went looking for a different recipe to use bananas and found this one.

¾ cup (75 g) unsalted pecans

¼ cup (56 g) unsalted margarine

⅓ cup (75 g) plus ¼ cup (60 g) brown sugar, divided

2 cups (250 g) flour

1 tablespoon (13.8 g) baking powder

6 tablespoons (90 ml) applesauce

⅔ cup (150 g) mashed bananas

Preheat oven to 375°F (190°C, or gas mark 5). Divide pecans, margarine, and ⅓ cup (75 g) brown sugar between 12 muffin cups. Bake for 5 minutes, or until margarine is melted. Combine flour and baking powder. Stir in applesauce and banana until mixture forms a soft dough. On a lightly floured surface, knead dough a few times until it holds together. Roll or press dough into a 9 × 12-inch (23 × 30-cm) rectangle. Spread remaining ¼ cup (60 g) brown sugar over dough. Roll up from long side. Slice into 12 rolls. Place each in a muffin cup. Bake for 12 to 15 minutes, or until golden. Allow to cool 1 minute before inverting onto a serving platter.

—
Yield: 12 servings

PER SERVING: 212 calories (37% from fat, 6% from protein, 58% from carbohydrate); 3 g protein; 9 g total fat; 1 g saturated fat; 5 g monounsaturated fat; 2 g polyunsaturated fat; 31 g carbohydrate; 2 g fiber; 13 g sugar; 75 mg phosphorus; 89 mg calcium; 2 mg iron; 168 mg sodium; 142 mg potassium; 214 IU vitamin A; 46 mg ATE vitamin E; 1 mg vitamin C; 0 mg cholesterol; 20 g water

Reduced-Fat Biscuits

This is a basic biscuit recipe, to which you could add other herbs and spices, a little low fat cheese, or whatever strikes your fancy. They can be made as drop biscuits as well as the rolled and cut version described below.

2 cups (250 g) flour

4 teaspoons (18.4 g) baking powder

2 teaspoons (8 g) sugar

½ teaspoon (1.5 g) cream of tartar

¼ cup (56 g) unsalted margarine

⅔ cup (160 ml) skim milk

Preheat oven to 450°F (230°C, or gas mark 8). Stir together flour, baking powder, sugar, and cream of tartar. Cut in margarine until mixture resembles coarse crumbs. Add milk. Stir until just mixed. Knead gently on a floured surface a few times. Press to ½-inch (1.3-cm) thickness. Cut out with a 2½-inch (6.3-cm) biscuit cutter. Transfer to an ungreased baking sheet. Bake for 10 to 12 minutes, or until golden brown.

—

Yield: 10 servings

PER SERVING: 142 calories (30% from fat, 9% from protein, 60% from carbohydrate); 3 g protein; 5 g total fat; 1 g saturated fat; 3 g monounsaturated fat; 1 g polyunsaturated fat; 21 g carbohydrate; 1 g fiber; 1 g sugar; 89 mg phosphorus; 139 mg calcium; 1 mg iron; 255 mg sodium; 87 mg potassium; 273 IU vitamin A; 65 mg ATE vitamin E; 0 mg vitamin C; 0 mg cholesterol; 19 g water

TIP

If you don't have a biscuit cutter, you can use a drinking glass or just cut the dough into squares with a knife.

Whole Wheat Biscuits

A small variation of the standard biscuit recipe. I sometimes add a little dill to them. If you don't have a biscuit cutter, you can use a drinking glass or just cut it into squares with a knife.

1½ cups (188 g) flour

½ cup (60 g) whole wheat flour

2 teaspoons (8 g) sugar

1 tablespoons (13.8 g) baking powder

¼ cup (56 g) unsalted margarine

⅔ cup (160 ml) skim milk

Preheat oven to 450°F (230°C, or gas mark 8). Stir together flours, sugar, and baking powder. Cut in margarine until mixture resembles coarse crumbs. Add milk. Stir until just mixed. Knead gently on a floured surface a few times. Press to ½-inch (1.3-cm) thickness. Cut out with a 2½-inch (6.3-cm) biscuit cutter. Transfer to an ungreased baking sheet. Bake for 10 to 12 minutes, or until golden brown.

—
Yield: 10 servings

PER SERVING: 141 calories (30% from fat, 10% from protein, 60% from carbohydrate); 4 g protein; 5 g total fat; 1 g saturated fat; 3 g monounsaturated fat; 1 g polyunsaturated fat; 22 g carbohydrate; 1 g fiber; 1 g sugar; 153 mg phosphorus; 275 mg calcium; 2 mg iron; 498 mg sodium; 80 mg potassium; 274 IU vitamin A; 65 mg ATE vitamin E; 0 mg vitamin C; 0 mg cholesterol; 19 g water

Lower-Fat Restaurant-Style Biscuits

This recipe has the flakiness and the buttery flavor typical of biscuits served at fast-food chicken restaurants, but without the fat and sodium.

2 cups (250 g) flour

1 tablespoon (13.8 g) baking powder

4 tablespoons (56 g) unsalted margarine, divided

2 ounces (55 g) fat-free sour cream

½ cup (120 ml) club soda, at room temperature

Preheat oven to 375°F (190°C, or gas mark 5). Stir flour and baking powder together. Cut in 2 tablespoons (28 g) margarine with a pastry blender or two knives until mixture resembles coarse crumbs. Mix sour cream and club soda into flour mixture. Turn out onto a lightly floured surface and knead lightly. Roll or pat to ½-inch (1.3-cm) thickness. Cut into 6 biscuits with a biscuit cutter or sharp knife. Place biscuits in an 8 × 8-inch (20 × 20-cm) baking dish sprayed with nonstick vegetable oil spray. Melt remaining margarine and pour over the top. Bake for 20 to 25 minutes, or until golden brown.

—
Yield: 6 servings

PER SERVING: 232 calories (32% from fat, 9% from protein, 59% from carbohydrate); 5 g protein; 8 g total fat; 2 g saturated fat; 4 g monounsaturated fat; 1 g polyunsaturated fat; 33 g carbohydrate; 1 g fiber; 0 g sugar; 109 mg phosphorus; 158 mg calcium; 2 mg iron; 335 mg sodium; 66 mg potassium; 435 IU vitamin A; 101 mg ATE vitamin E; 0 mg vitamin C; 4 mg cholesterol; 34 g water

Lower-Fat Cornbread

Cornbread goes well with a lot of things. I've found here, like with a lot of recipes, that reducing the amount of fat called for doesn't really affect the end product at all.

1 cup (140 g) cornmeal

1 cup (125 g) flour

¼ cup (50 g) sugar

1 tablespoon (13.8 g) baking powder

2 tablespoons (28 g) unsalted margarine

1 cup (235 ml) skim milk

¼ cup (60 ml) egg substitute

Preheat oven to 425°F (220°C, or gas mark 7). Mix together cornmeal, flour, sugar, and baking powder. Cut in margarine until mixture resembles coarse crumbs. Stir milk and egg substitute together and add to dry ingredients, stirring until just mixed. Place in a 9-inch (23-cm) square pan sprayed with nonstick vegetable oil spray and bake for 20 to 25 minutes.

—
Yield: 12 servings

PER SERVING: 133 calories (17% from fat, 11% from protein, 73% from carbohydrate); 4 g protein; 2 g total fat; 1 g saturated fat; 1 g monounsaturated fat; 0 g polyunsaturated fat; 24 g carbohydrate; 1 g fiber; 4 g sugar; 81 mg phosphorus; 103 mg calcium; 1 mg iron; 165 mg sodium; 88 mg potassium; 189 IU vitamin A; 35 mg ATE vitamin E; 0 mg vitamin C; 0 mg cholesterol; 26 g water

Oatmeal Pancakes

A nice change for Sunday morning breakfast.

1¼ cups (285 ml) skim milk

1 cup (80 g) quick-cooking oats

½ cup (120 ml) egg substitute

½ cup (60 g) whole wheat flour

1 tablespoon (15 g) brown sugar

1 teaspoon (2.3 g) cinnamon

1 tablespoon (13.8 g) baking powder

Combine milk and oats in a bowl and let stand 5 minutes. Add egg substitute and mix well. Add remaining ingredients and stir until just blended. Cook on a hot griddle, turning when bubbles form on the tops of the pancakes and burst. Flip pancakes and finish cooking on the other side.

—
Yield: 6 servings

PER SERVING: 135 calories (12% from fat, 23% from protein, 65% from carbohydrate); 8 g protein; 2 g total fat; 0 g saturated fat; 1 g monounsaturated fat; 1 g polyunsaturated fat; 22 g carbohydrate; 3 g fiber; 3 g sugar; 232 mg phosphorus; 237 mg calcium; 2 mg iron; 313 mg sodium; 260 mg potassium; 181 IU vitamin A; 31 mg ATE vitamin E; 1 mg vitamin C; 1 mg cholesterol; 66 g water

11

Slightly Healthy Sweets

The story of most desserts is similar to the one for quick breads: They often contain more fat than they need to. In this chapter you'll find a number of healthier options to satisfy your sweet tooth. It includes not just lower-fat versions of cakes and cookies, but also some naturally healthy things that you may not normally consider, like cobblers and fruit desserts.

Low Fat Cranberry Cake

When I first came across a version of this recipe it sounded so good that I had to try it. Of course, the original was full of fat and sodium, but we've solved that problem with no loss of taste.

2 cups (220 g) cranberries

1¾ cups (350 g) sugar, divided

½ cup (120 ml) water

1 cup (125 g) flour

1½ teaspoons (7 g) baking powder

½ cup (120 ml) applesauce

¼ cup (60 ml) egg substitute

¼ cup (60 ml) skim milk

¼ cup (60 ml) orange juice

1 teaspoon (1.7 g) orange peel, grated

½ teaspoon (3 ml) vanilla

—
Yield: 12 servings

Preheat oven to 375°F (190°C, or gas mark 5). Spray bottom and sides of a 9-inch (23-cm) round baking pan with nonstick vegetable oil spray. Combine cranberries, 1 cup (200 g) sugar, and water in a large saucepan. Bring to a boil. Reduce heat and simmer for 10 minutes, or until slightly thickened to a syrupy consistency. Pour into prepared pan. Cool to room temperature. Sift together flour, remaining ¾ cup (150 g) sugar, and baking powder into a large bowl. In another bowl, stir applesauce, egg substitute, milk, orange juice, orange peel, and vanilla until blended. Stir into dry ingredients just until blended. Pour over cranberry mixture. Bake for 25 to 30 minutes, or until a wooden pick inserted in the center comes out clean. Let cake cool in pan about 5 minutes. Loosen cake around edges of pan. Place inverted serving platter over cake and turn both upside down. Shake gently, then remove pan. Serve warm.

PER SERVING: 232 calories (2% from fat, 3% from protein, 94% from carbohydrate); 2 g protein; 1 g total fat; 0 g saturated fat; 0 g monounsaturated fat; 0 g polyunsaturated fat; 57 g carbohydrate; 2 g fiber; 44 g sugar; 39 mg phosphorus; 49 mg calcium; 1 mg iron; 75 mg sodium; 64 mg potassium; 35 IU vitamin A; 3 mg ATE vitamin E; 2 mg vitamin C; 0 mg cholesterol; 37 g water

Low Fat Devil's Food Cake

This makes a fairly heavy, very moist cake, almost like brownies or bars.

2 cups (250 g) flour

1¾ cups (350 g) sugar

½ cup (43 g) unsweetened cocoa powder

1 tablespoon (13.8 g) baking soda

⅔ cup (160 ml) applesauce

⅓ cup (80 ml) buttermilk

2 tablespoons (30 ml) canola oil

1 cup (235 ml) coffee

Preheat oven to 350°F (180°C, or gas mark 4). Spray a 9 × 13-inch (23 × 33-cm) pan with nonstick vegetable oil spray and then dust with flour, shaking out the excess. In a large bowl, mix together flour, sugar, cocoa, and baking soda. Stir in applesauce, buttermilk, and oil. Heat coffee to boiling and stir into batter. Batter will be thin. Pour into prepared pan. Bake for 35 to 40 minutes, or until a wooden pick inserted in the center comes out clean.

—
Yield: 24 servings

PER SERVING: 116 calories (12% from fat, 5% from protein, 83% from carbohydrate); 2 g protein; 2 g total fat; 0 g saturated fat; 1 g monounsaturated fat; 0 g polyunsaturated fat; 25 g carbohydrate; 1 g fiber; 16 g sugar; 28 mg phosphorus; 8 mg calcium; 1 mg iron; 162 mg sodium; 55 mg potassium; 2 IU vitamin A; 0 mg ATE vitamin E; 0 mg vitamin C; 0 mg cholesterol; 20 g water

Lower-Fat Carrot Cake

This is lighter than most carrot cakes, but the flavor is very close to the traditional one.

¼ cup (60 ml) canola oil

¾ cup (180 ml) applesauce

½ cup (120 ml) skim milk

1½ cups (300 g) sugar

¾ cup (180 ml) egg substitute

2 cups (250 g) flour

4 teaspoons (18.4 g) baking soda

2½ teaspoons (5.8 g) cinnamon

½ teaspoon (1.1 g) nutmeg

½ teaspoon (1.2 g) ground cloves

1½ teaspoons (8 ml) vanilla

2 cups (260 g) shredded carrot

½ cup (60 g) chopped walnuts

½ cup (80 g) raisins

8 ounces (225 g) crushed pineapple, undrained

Preheat oven to 350°F (180°C, or gas mark 4). Coat a rectangular 9 × 13-inch (23 × 33-cm) cake pan with nonstick vegetable oil spray. In one bowl, beat together oil, applesauce, milk, sugar, and egg substitute. In another bowl, stir together flour, baking soda, cinnamon, nutmeg, and cloves. Combine both sets of ingredients and beat, mixing in vanilla. Add carrots, walnuts, raisins, and pineapple, mixing well after each addition. Bake for 1 hour, or until done. Cool and remove from pan.

—

Yield: 16 servings

PER SERVING: 239 calories (24% from fat, 8% from protein, 68% from carbohydrate); 5 g protein; 7 g total fat; 1 g saturated fat; 3 g monounsaturated fat; 3 g polyunsaturated fat; 42 g carbohydrate; 2 g fiber; 27 g sugar; 73 mg phosphorus; 37 mg calcium; 1 mg iron; 353 mg sodium; 206 mg potassium; 2757 IU vitamin A; 5 mg ATE vitamin E; 3 mg vitamin C; 0 mg cholesterol; 55 g water

Apple Crunch

An easy-to-put-together apple dessert that satisfies without having too much fat.

FOR APPLES:

4 apples, peeled, cored, and chopped

½ cup (100 g) sugar

1 teaspoon (2.3 g) cinnamon

1 tablespoon (14 g) unsalted margarine

FOR TOPPING:

½ cup (60 g) flour

½ cup (100 g) sugar

1 teaspoon (4.6 g) baking powder

¼ cup (60 ml) egg substitute

½ cup (100 g) sugar

1 tablespoon (14 g) unsalted margarine

TO MAKE THE APPLES: Preheat oven to 350°F (180°C, or gas mark 4). Mix apples, sugar, and cinnamon; pour into a greased 8 × 8-inch (20 × 20-cm) baking dish. Dot with margarine.

TO MAKE THE TOPPING: Mix topping ingredients and pour over apples. Bake for 30 to 35 minutes.

—
Yield: 6 servings

PER SERVING: 317 calories (12% from fat, 3% from protein, 85% from carbohydrate); 3 g protein; 4 g total fat; 1 g saturated fat; 2 g monounsaturated fat; 1 g polyunsaturated fat; 70 g carbohydrate; 2 g fiber; 59 g sugar; 53 mg phosphorus; 65 mg calcium; 1 mg iron; 141 mg sodium; 130 mg potassium; 271 IU vitamin A; 46 mg ATE vitamin E; 4 mg vitamin C; 0 mg cholesterol; 85 g water

Crumb-Topped Cherry Cobbler

A quick and easy cobbler recipe, low in fat.

21-ounce (595-g) can cherry
pie filling

2 tablespoons (28 g) unsalted
margarine

½ cup (40 g) quick-cooking oats

¼ cup (30 g) flour

½ cup (100 g) sugar

2 tablespoons (16 g) chopped
pecans

Preheat oven to 350°F (180°C, or gas mark 4). Spray a 2-quart (1.9-L) casserole dish with nonstick vegetable oil spray. Pour cherry pie filling into prepared dish. Mix margarine, oats, flour, sugar, and pecans. Crumble over cherry pie filling. Bake for 20 to 25 minutes.

—
Yield: 8 servings

PER SERVING: 205 calories (19% from fat, 3% from protein, 77% from carbohydrate); 2 g protein; 4 g total fat; 1 g saturated fat; 2 g monounsaturated fat; 1 g polyunsaturated fat; 40 g carbohydrate; 1 g fiber; 13 g sugar; 46 mg phosphorus; 15 mg calcium; 1 mg iron; 44 mg sodium; 111 mg potassium; 303 IU vitamin A; 34 mg ATE vitamin E; 3 mg vitamin C; 0 mg cholesterol; 55 g water

Strawberry Pie Filling

This comes from my mother, who sent it to me when she heard we'd been berry picking.

3 cups (510 g) strawberries, sliced

one prepared pie crust

1 cup (235 ml) water

2 tablespoons (16 g) cornstarch

½ cup (100 g) sugar

one 3-ounce (85 g) box sugar-free strawberry gelatin

Put sliced berries in pie crust. Combine water, cornstarch, and sugar. Heat until sugar is melted and mixture is clear. Stir in gelatin and pour over berries. Chill until set.

—
Yield: 8 servings

PER SERVING: 79 calories (2% from fat, 5% from protein, 93% from carbohydrate); 1 g protein; 0 g total fat; 0 g saturated fat; 0 g monounsaturated fat; 0 g polyunsaturated fat; 19 g carbohydrate; 1 g fiber; 15 g sugar; 30 mg phosphorus; 10 mg calcium; 0 mg iron; 4 mg sodium; 88 mg potassium; 7 IU vitamin A; 0 mg ATE vitamin E; 34 mg vitamin C; 0 mg cholesterol; 82 g water

TIP

The sugar-free gelatin has quite a bit less sodium than the regular kind.

Sweet Potato Pie

You'll be hard pressed to tell the difference between this and pumpkin pie.

FOR CRUST:

⅓ cup (80 ml) canola oil

1⅓ cups (165 g) flour

2 tablespoons (30 ml) cold water

FOR FILLING:

2 cups (650 g) cooked and mashed sweet potatoes

¾ cup (150 g) sugar

½ teaspoon (0.9 g) ground ginger

½ teaspoon (1.1 g) nutmeg

½ teaspoon (1.2 g) cinnamon

½ cup (120 ml) egg substitute

1½ cups (355 ml) fat-free evaporated milk

1 teaspoon (5 ml) vanilla

Preheat oven to 400°F (200°C, or gas mark 6).

TO MAKE THE CRUST: Add oil to flour and mix well with a fork. Sprinkle water over and mix well. With your hands, press dough into a ball and flatten. Roll between two pieces of waxed paper. Remove the top piece of waxed paper, invert over pie plate, and remove the other piece of waxed paper. Press into place.

TO MAKE THE FILLING: Combine sweet potatoes, sugar, ginger, nutmeg, and cinnamon in a mixing bowl. Add egg substitute and mix well. Add milk and vanilla and combine. Pour into pie shell. Bake for 45 to 50 minutes, or until knife inserted near the center comes out clean.

—
Yield: 8 servings

PER SERVING: 345 calories (26% from fat, 10% from protein, 64% from carbohydrate); 9 g protein; 10 g total fat; 1 g saturated fat; 3 g monounsaturated fat; 5 g polyunsaturated fat; 55 g carbohydrate; 3 g fiber; 29 g sugar; 162 mg phosphorus; 175 mg calcium; 2 mg iron; 106 mg sodium; 426 mg potassium; 13153 IU vitamin A; 57 mg ATE vitamin E; 11 mg vitamin C; 2 mg cholesterol; 123 g water

Meringue Cookies

These might just be the ultimate in fat-free cookies. They are such crunchy, sweet little nuggets that you won't even miss the fat.

3 egg whites

¼ teaspoon (0.8 g) cream of tartar

¾ cup (150 g) superfine sugar

Preheat oven to 225°F (110°C). Beat egg whites with an electric mixer on medium speed until foamy. Add cream of tartar and continue beating egg whites until soft peaks form. Gradually add sugar, beating well after each addition. Mix until all the sugar has been added and the egg whites are stiff and glossy. Drop by the tablespoon onto a baking sheet. Bake for 1 hour. Switch off oven and leave cookies in the oven for 2 to 3 hours.

—
Yield: 24 servings

PER SERVING: 17 calories (1% from fat, 11% from protein, 89% from carbohydrate); 0 g protein; 0 g total fat; 0 g saturated fat; 0 g monounsaturated fat; 0 g polyunsaturated fat; 4 g carbohydrate; 0 g fiber; 4 g sugar; 1 mg phosphorus; 0 mg calcium; 0 mg iron; 7 mg sodium; 12 mg potassium; 0 IU vitamin A; 0 mg ATE vitamin E; 0 mg vitamin C; 0 mg cholesterol; 4 g water

TIP

If you can't find superfine sugar, process regular sugar in a blender or food processor until it is powdery.

Thumbprint Cookies

These are wonderful cookies that no one will ever know are low in fat.

¼ cup (56 g) unsalted margarine, softened

½ cup (115 g) packed brown sugar

¼ cup (60 ml) egg substitute

1 teaspoon (5 ml) vanilla

1½ cups (185 g) flour

6 tablespoons (90 ml) raspberry jam

Preheat oven to 350°F (180°C, or gas mark 4). In a large bowl, cream margarine and brown sugar together using an electric mixer. Add egg substitute and vanilla, and mix until blended. Gradually add flour and mix, forming a large ball. Form 1-inch (2.5-cm) balls and place them 1 inch (2.5-cm) apart on a baking sheet, making a deep thumbprint in the center of each. Bake for 10 minutes. Remove from oven. After 1 minute, place on a wire rack to cool. Place 1 teaspoon (5 ml) of raspberry jam in the center of each cookie.

—

Yield: 24 servings

PER SERVING: 79 calories (23% from fat, 6% from protein, 71% from carbohydrate); 1 g protein; 2 g total fat; 0 g saturated fat; 1 g monounsaturated fat; 1 g polyunsaturated fat; 14 g carbohydrate; 0 g fiber; 7 g sugar; 14 mg phosphorus; 8 mg calcium; 1 mg iron; 8 mg sodium; 38 mg potassium; 93 IU vitamin A; 18 mg ATE vitamin E; 0 mg vitamin C; 0 mg cholesterol; 5 g water

Chocolate Chip Cookies

These are lighter than most chocolate chip cookies, owing to the beaten egg white. But the taste will satisfy any cookie lover.

2¼ cups (280 g) flour

1 teaspoon (4.6 g) baking powder

¾ cup (170 g) brown sugar, packed

2 tablespoons (28 g) unsalted margarine

1 teaspoon (5 ml) vanilla extract

4 large egg whites, room temperature

½ cup (100 g) sugar

⅓ cup (80 ml) light corn syrup

1¼ cups (220 g) semisweet chocolate chips

—

Yield: 48 servings

Preheat oven to 375°F (190°C, or gas mark 5). Lightly spoon flour into dry measuring cups and level with a knife. Combine flour and baking powder. Beat brown sugar, margarine, and vanilla extract with an electric mixer on medium speed for 5 minutes, or until well-blended. Beat egg whites until foamy using clean, dry beaters. Gradually add sugar, 1 tablespoon at a time; beat until soft peaks form. Add corn syrup; beat until stiff peaks form. Fold brown sugar mixture into egg white mixture. Add flour mixture and stir to combine. Drop dough by level tablespoons 1 inch (2.5 cm) apart onto baking sheets coated with nonstick vegetable oil spray. Bake for 10 minutes, or until golden. Remove from the oven and let stand 5 minutes. Remove cookies from pans, and cool on wire racks. Store loosely covered.

PER SERVING: 76 calories (21% from fat, 6% from protein, 73% from carbohydrate); 1 g protein; 2 g total fat; 1 g saturated fat; 1 g monounsaturated fat; 0 g polyunsaturated fat; 15 g carbohydrate; 0 g fiber; 8 g sugar; 16 mg phosphorus; 12 mg calcium; 0 mg iron; 23 mg sodium; 39 mg potassium; 25 IU vitamin A; 6 mg ATE vitamin E; 0 mg vitamin C; 0 mg cholesterol; 4 g water

Pumpkin Cookies

These cookies sometimes end up being eaten for breakfast around our house. They are almost like muffins, only smaller.

2 cups (250 g) flour

1 teaspoon (4.6 g) baking powder

½ teaspoon (2.3 g) baking soda

1 teaspoon (2.3 g) cinnamon

½ teaspoon (0.9 g) ground ginger

1 teaspoon (1.9 g) ground allspice

¼ cup (60 ml) canola oil

1 cup (225 g) packed brown sugar

6 tablespoons (90 ml) egg substitute

1 cup (225 g) canned or cooked
fresh pumpkin

1 teaspoon (5 ml) vanilla

Preheat oven to 350°F (180°C, or gas mark 4). In a medium bowl, combine flour, baking powder, baking soda, cinnamon, ginger, and allspice. In a large bowl beat oil, brown sugar, egg substitute, pumpkin, and vanilla. Stir flour mixture into wet ingredients until just combined. Drop spoonfuls of dough about 1 inch (2.5 cm) apart on an ungreased baking sheet. Bake for 12 to 14 minutes.

—
Yield: 30 servings

PER SERVING: 81 calories (23% from fat, 7% from protein, 70% from carbohydrate); 1 g protein; 2 g total fat; 0 g saturated fat; 1 g monounsaturated fat; 1 g polyunsaturated fat; 14 g carbohydrate; 1 g fiber; 7 g sugar; 21 mg phosphorus; 22 mg calcium; 1 mg iron; 46 mg sodium; 63 mg potassium; 1283 IU vitamin A; 0 mg ATE vitamin E; 0 mg vitamin C; 0 mg cholesterol; 11 g water

About the Author

After being diagnosed with congestive heart failure, Dick Logue threw himself into the process of creating healthy versions of his favorite recipes. A cook since the age of twelve, Logue grows his own vegetables, bakes his own bread, and cans a variety of foods. He currently has a website, www.lowsodiumcooking.com, and his weekly online newsletter, complete with the latest recipes and tips, is read by more than 17,000 people. He lives on a little farm in the woods of southern Maryland with his wife, Ginger, two of their three children, and an assortment of animals.

Index